Midwifery Casebook for PB BSc Nursing

Midwifery Casebook for PB BSc Nursing

As per INC Syllabus

Gowri Sayee Jagadesan
Professor and HOD
Department of Obstetrics and Gynecological Nursing
Fortis Institute of Nursing
Bengaluru, Karnataka, India

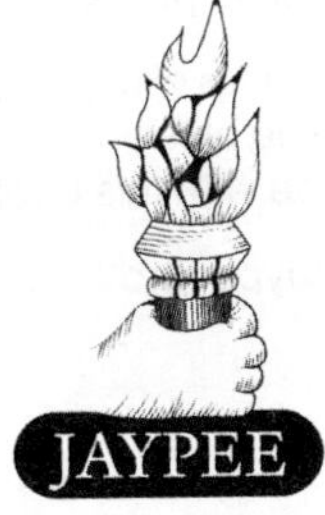

JAYPEE

JAYPEE BROTHERS MEDICAL PUBLISHERS

The Health Sciences Publisher

New Delhi | London

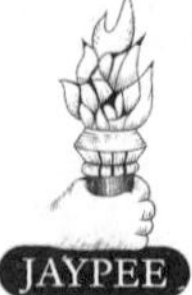

Jaypee Brothers Medical Publishers (P) Ltd

Headquarters
EMCA House
23/23-B, Ansari Road, Daryaganj
New Delhi - 110 002, India
Landline: +91-11-23272143, +91-11-23272703
+91-11-23282021, +91-11-23245672
E-mail: jaypee@jaypeebrothers.com

Corporate Office
4838/24, Ansari Road, Daryaganj
New Delhi - 110 002, India
Phone: +91-11-43574357
Fax: +91-11-43574314
E-mail: jaypee@jaypeebrothers.com

Overseas Office
J.P. Medical Ltd
83 Victoria Street, London
SW1H 0HW (UK)
Phone: +44 20 3170 8910
E-mail: info@jpmedpub.com

EU GPSR Authorised Representative
Logos Europe, 9 rue Nicolas Poussin
17000, La Rochelle, France
Phone: +33 (0) 6 67 93 73 78
E-mail: contact@logoseurope.eu

Website: www.jaypeebrothers.com
Website: www.jaypeedigital.com

Inquiries for bulk sales may be solicited at: jaypee@jaypeebrothers.com

Midwifery Casebook for PB BSc Nursing

First Edition: **2020,** Reprint: 2023, 2024, **2026**

ISBN: 978-93-86261-81-6

Printed at: Samrat Offset Pvt. Ltd.

Dedicated to
all the women, mothers and midwives

Respect A Woman Because

You can feel her INNOCENCE in the form of a daughter
You can feel her CARE in the form of a sister
You can feel her WARMTH in the form of a friend
You can feel her PASSION in the form of a beloved
You can feel her DEDICATION in the form of a wife
You can feel her DIVINITY in the form of a mother
You can feel her BLESSING in the form of a grandmother
Yet she is so TOUGH too
Her heart is so TENDER... So NAUGHTY... So CHARMING...
So SHARING... So MELODIUS... She is a WOMAN..
And She is LIFE!!!

To all the wonderful women.

A **Mother** is she, who can take the place of all others, but whose place no one else can take.

Midwives are truly the unsung heroines of the challenge to reduce the risks of the women face in bringing forth life.

Preface

Midwifery Casebook for PB BSc Nursing provides a broad-based knowledge aimed to build upon the skills and competencies acquired at the Diploma in Nursing level. It is specifically directed to the upgrading of critical thinking skills, competencies and standards required for practice of professional nursing and midwifery.

This casebook is designed as per the clinical requirements of 1st year PB BSc (N), Maternal Nursing.

The key features of this book are:

- Helps the midwifery students in completing their clinical requirements as per the revised INC syllabus
- Helps also in collecting the specific and relevant information related to the different components of maternal nursing
- Provides formats for entering the data in a systematic manner
- Also provides comprehensive care to the mother during her antenatal, intranatal and postnatal period including the newborn baby
- Helps the students to gain adequate knowledge and specific skills related to maternal nursing
- Also helps the clinical instructors to guide the students in their daily clinical practices.

Gowri Sayee Jagadesan

Acknowledgments

The most important aspect in every human life is to trust God in every circumstance. I thank God Almighty for His abundant blessings showered on me to complete this casebook successfully.

It is my privilege to extend my prime thanks to my parents who made me to study this wonderful subject.

My heartfelt thanks to my husband who is the real motivator for my professional growth and also to my children for their love and support.

Genuine gratitude and heartfelt thanks to Prof Prabhuswamy AC, Principal, Fortis Institute of Nursing, who is the real architect of this casebook for helping me in constructing and designing this book.

I express my deep sense of gratitude to Prof Shridhar KV, Principal, Adesh College of Nursing, Adesh University, Punjab, India for introducing me to Mr Santhosh, Commissioning Editor of M/s Jaypee Brothers Medical Publishers (P) Ltd; I also thank Mr Santosh for his constant and enormous support in all the way for completion of this casebook.

My heartfelt thanks to Mrs Sabitha Sibbala (Associate Professor), Mrs Sophia (Assistant Lecturer) and Ms Divya (Assistant Lecturer), Department of Obstetrics and Gynecology for their valuable suggestions related to the theoretical and practical components of maternal nursing.

I am grateful to all my colleagues for their continuous motivation, support and encouragement.

INC Syllabus

MATERNAL NURSING

Placement: First year

Time Allotted: Theory—60 hours
Practical—240 hours

COURSE DESCRIPTION

This course is designed to widen the student's knowledge of obstetrics during pregnancy, labor and puerperium. It also helps acquire knowledge and develop skill in rendering optimum nursing care to a childbearing mother in a hospital or community and help in the management of common gynecological problems.

OBJECTIVES

At end of the course, the student will:
- Describe the physiology of pregnancy, labor and puerperium.
- Manage normal pregnancy, labor and puerperium.
- Explain the physiology of lactation and advice on management of breastfeeding.
- Be skilled in providing pre- and postoperative nursing care in obstetric conditions.
- Identify and manage high-risk pregnancy, including appropriate referrals.
- Propagate the concept and motivate acceptance of family planning methods.
- Teach, guide and supervise auxiliary midwifery personnel.

COURSE CONTENTS

UNIT I

Introduction and historical review
Planned parenthood
Maternal morbidity and mortality rates
Legislations related to maternity benefits, MTP Act, incentives for family planning, etc.

UNIT II

Review of the anatomy and physiology of female reproductive system
Female pelvis (normal and contracted)
Review of fetal development

UNIT III

Physiology of pregnancy
Signs and symptoms and diagnosis of pregnancy
Antenatal care, management of pregnancy, labor and puerperium
Pregnant women with HIV/AIDS
Management of common gynecological problems

UNIT IV

The newborn baby
Care of the baby at birth including resuscitation
Essential newborn care
Feeding

Jaundice and infection
Small and large for date babies
Intensive care of the newborn
Trauma and hemorrhage

UNIT V

Management of abnormal pregnancy, labor and puerperium
Abortion, ectopic pregnancy and vesicular mole
Pregnancy-induced hypertension, gestational diabetes, anemia, heart disease
Urinary infections, antepartum hemorrhage
Abnornal labor (malposition and malpresentation)
Uterine inertia
Disorders of puerperium
Management of engorged breast, cracked nipples, breast abscess and mastitis
Pueperal sepsis
Postpartum hemorrhage
Inversion and prolapse of uterus, obstetrical emergencies
Obstetrical procedures, i.e. forceps, vacuum, episiotomy, cesarean section

UNIT VI

Drugs in obstetrics
Effects of drugs during pregnancy, labor and puerperium on mother and baby

UNIT VII

National Welfare Programs for Women
National Family Welfare Program
Infertile couple
Problems associated with unwanted pregnancy
Unwed mothers

PRACTICUM

1. The students will:
    a. Be posted in antenatal clinic, MCH clinic, antenatal ward, labor room, postnatal ward, maternity OT, MTP room.
    b. Visit welfare agencies for women and write observation report.
    c. Follow nursing process in providing care to 3–6 patients.
    d. Write at least two nursing care studies and do a presentation.
    e. Give at least one planned health teaching to a group of mothers.
2. Practice following nursing procedures.
    a. Antenatal and postnatal examination, per vaginal examination
    b. Conduct normal delivery, stitching of episiotomy (for male candidates minimum conduct of 5 deliveries).
    c. Motivation of family for adopting family planning methods.
    d. Motivate family for planned parenthood.
    e. Assist in various diagnostic and therapeutic procedures including IUD insertion and removal.

Contents

Midwifery Casebook for PC BSc Nursing

Name of the Student (in Block Letters) : ....

Register No. : ....

Age and Date of Birth : ....

Year : ....

Date of Joining the Course : ....

Passport size photograph

Name and Address of the Institution : ....

....

....

....

....

Name of the Hospital/Nursing Home : ....

....

....

Signature of Student	Signature of Class Coordinator	Signature of HOD	Signature of Principal
Date:	Date:	Date:	Date:

CHAPTER 1

Antenatal Examination

ANTENATAL EXAMINATION PERFORMED

Sl No.	Register No.	Name of the Mother	Date of Examination	Age	Obstetrical Score	LMP*	EDD†	Gestational Age (in weeks)	Fundal Height (cm)	Abdominal Girth (cm)	Findings	FHS‡	General Condition of the Mother						Other investigations and findings	Treatment and Advice Given
													Weight (kg)	Height (cm)	Blood Group	BP§ (mm Hg)	Urine			
																	Albumin	Sugar		
1.																				
2.																				
3.																				
4.																				
5.																				
6.																				
7.																				
8.																				
9.																				
10.																				

*LMP, last menstrual period; †EDD, Expected date of delivery; ‡FHS, Fetal heart sound; §BP, blood pressure.

ANTENATAL EXAMINATION (1)

HISTORY COLLECTION

1. Baseline Data:

Name of the Mother: ....

Date of Registration: ....

Age: ....

Date of Admission: ....

Religion: ....

Date of Assessment: ....

Hospital Number: ....

Procedure Performed: ....

[Wards, Primary health center (PHC), Out patient department (OPD), Home]

Marital Status: ....

LMP: ....

EDD: ....

Period of gestation: ....

Obstetrical score:

G		P		L		A		S		D	

G-Gravida: ....

P-Para: ....

L-Living: ....

A-Abortion: ....

S-Still birth: ....

D-Death: ....

Diagnosis: ....

Address: ....

2. Socioeconomic History:

Educational Status: ....

Husband: ....

Wife: ....

Occupation: ....

Husband: ....

Wife: ....

Total income: ....

Type of house: ....

Living standard:

Ownership of the house: Own house/Rented house

Lighting facility: ....

Environmental conditions of the house:

Water facility: ....

Toilet facility: ....

Drainage, kitchen, garden: ....

Pet animals: ....

Cultural background: ....

3. Family History:

Sl No.	*Name of the Family Member*	*Age*	*Sex*	*Educational Status*	*Occupation*	*Relationship with the Mother*	*Health Status*
1.							
2.							
3.							
4.							
5.							
6.							

History of any

- Communicable diseases: ....
- Hereditary diseases: ....
- Twin pregnancy: ....
- Bad obstetrical history: ....

4. Personal History:
   - Dietary pattern: ....
   - Sleeping pattern: ....
   - Habits: ....
   - Bowel elimination: ....
   - Bladder elimination: ....
   - Immunization history: ....
   - Sexual history: ....
   - Drug history/Drug allergy: ....

5. Menstrual History: ....

....

6. Marital History: ....

....

7. Contraceptive History: ....

....

8. Previous Medical and Surgical History: ....

....

9. Previous Obstetrical History:

Sl No.	*Year*	*Antenatal Period*	*Intranatal Period*	*Postnatal Period*	*Alive/ Stillbirth*	*Sex*	*Weight*	*Remarks*
1								
2								
3								
4								
5								
6								

10. Present Obstetrical History:

    a. Antenatal: ....

    ....

    ....

    b. Intranatal: ....

    ....

    ....

    c. Postnatal: ....

    ....

    ....

ANTENATAL EXAMINATION

1. General Examination:

General appearance: .... Psychological status: ....

Head: .... Hair: ....

Facial appearance: .... Eyes: ....

Ears: .... Nose: ....

Mouth: .... Mucus membranes: ....

Gums: .... Teeth: ....

Tongue: .... Tonsils: ....

Neck: .... Upper limbs: ....

Chest: .... Lungs: ....

Heart: .... Lower limbs: ....

Back: ....

Vital signs:

Temperature: .... Pulse: ....

Respiration: .... Blood pressure: ....

2. Obstetrical Examination:

a. Breast Examination:

Size and shape: .... Sensation: ....

Primary areola: .... Secondary areola: ....

Montgomery tubercles: .... Colostrums: ....

Nipples: ....

b. Abdominal Examination:

Inspection: ....

Size of the abdomen: .... Shape of the abdomen: ....

Contour of the abdominal wall:

- Skin changes on the abdomen: ....
- Previous operation scar: ....
- Striae gravidarum: ....
- Linea nigra: ....
- Umbilicus: Flattened/Protruded/Dimpled.

Visible fetal movement: ....

Flank region/Filled/Empty

Appearance of the skin infection: ....

Fundal Height (in cm): .... Abdominal girth (in cm): ....

- Abdominal palpation:

Fundal palpation: ....

Lateral palpation: ....

(i) Right lateral palpation: ....

(ii) Left lateral palpation: ....

Pelvic Palpation: ....

Pawlik's grip: ....

Auscultation: ....

- Findings:

Lie: .... Attitude: ....

Presentation: .... Position: ....

Denominator: ....

- Vaginal examination:

Discharge: ....

Sign of infection: .... Any other specify: ....

Investigation done:

Date	*Investigation Done*	*Mothers Value*	*Normal Value*	*Remarks*

Any other specific investigation: ....

- Treatment Given:

Name of the Drug	*Dosag/Route/Frequency*	*Action*	*Side Effects*	*Nurses Responsibility*

Sl No.	*Needs Identified*	*Nursing Care Given*

- Antenatal advices: ....
....
....
....
....

General health condition of the mother: ....

Signature of the Student

Signature of the Supervisor

ANTENATAL EXAMINATION (2)

HISTORY COLLECTION

1. Baseline Data:

   Name of the Mother: .... Date of Registration: ....

   Age: .... Date of Admission: ....

   Religion: .... Date of Assessment: ....

   Hospital Number: .... Procedure Performed: ....

   [Wards, Primary health center (PHC), Out patient department (OPD), Home]

   Marital Status: ....

   LMP: ....

   EDD: ....

   Period of gestation: ....

   Obstetrical score:

G		P		L		A		S		D	

   G-Gravida: .... P-Para: ....

   L-Living: .... A-Abortion: ....

   S-Still birth: .... D-Death: ....

   Diagnosis: ....

   Address: ....

2. Socioeconomic History:

   Educational Status: .... Husband: ....

   Wife: ....

   Occupation: .... Husband: ....

   Wife: ....

   Total income: ....

   Type of house: ....

   Living standard:

   Ownership of the house: Own house/Rented house

   Lighting facility: ....

   Environmental conditions of the house: Water facility: ....

   Toilet facility: ....

Drainage, kitchen, garden: ....

Pet animals: ....

Cultural background: ....

3. Family History:

Sl No.	Name of the Family Member	Age	Sex	Educational Status	Occupation	Relationship with the Mother	Health Status
1.							
2.							
3.							
4.							
5.							
6.							

History of any

- Communicable diseases: ....
- Hereditary diseases: ....
- Twin pregnancy: ....
- Bad obstetrical history: ....

4. Personal History:
   - Dietary pattern: ....
   - Sleeping pattern: ....
   - Habits: ....
   - Bowel elimination: ....
   - Bladder elimination: ....
   - Immunization history: ....
   - Sexual history: ....
   - Drug history/Drug allergy: ....

5. Menstrual History: ....

....

6. Marital History: ....

....

7. Contraceptive History: ....

....

8. Previous Medical and Surgical History: ....

....

9. Previous Obstetrical History:

Sl No.	*Year*	*Antenatal Period*	*Intranatal Period*	*Postnatal Period*	*Alive/ Stillbirth*	*Sex*	*Weight*	*Remarks*
1								
2								
3								
4								
5								
6								

10. Present Obstetrical History:

    a. Antenatal: ....

    ....

    ....

    b. Intranatal: ....

    ....

    ....

    c. Postnatal: ....

    ....

    ....

ANTENATAL EXAMINATION

1. General Examination:

   General appearance: .... Psychological status: ....

   Head: .... Hair: ....

   Facial appearance: .... Eyes: ....

   Ears: .... Nose: ....

   Mouth: .... Mucus membranes: ....

   Gums: .... Teeth: ....

   Tongue: .... Tonsils: ....

   Neck: .... Upper limbs: ....

   Chest: .... Lungs: ....

   Heart: .... Lower limbs: ....

   Back: ....

Vital signs:

   Temperature: .... Pulse: ....

   Respiration: .... Blood pressure: ....

2. Obstetrical Examination:

   a. Breast Examination:

      Size and shape: .... Sensation: ....

      Primary areola: .... Secondary areola: ....

      Montgomery tubercles: .... Colostrums: ....

      Nipples: ....

   b. Abdominal Examination:

      Inspection: ....

      Size of the abdomen: .... Shape of the abdomen: ....

      Contour of the abdominal wall:

      - Skin changes on the abdomen: ....
      - Previous operation scar: ....
      - Striae gravidarum: ....
      - Linea nigra: ....
      - Umbilicus: Flattened/Protruded/Dimpled.

        Visible fetal movement: ....

        Flank region/Filled/Empty

Appearance of the skin infection: ....

Fundal Height (in cm): .... Abdominal girth (in cm): ....

- Abdominal palpation:

Fundal palpation: ....

Lateral palpation: ....

(i) Right lateral palpation: ....

(ii) Left lateral palpation: ....

Pelvic Palpation: ....

Pawlik's grip: ....

Auscultation: ....

- Findings:

Lie: .... Attitude: ....

Presentation: .... Position: ....

- Vaginal examination:

Denominator: ....

Discharge: ....

Sign of infection: .... Any other specify: ....

Investigation done:

Date	*Investigation Done*	*Mothers Value*	*Normal Value*	*Remarks*

Any other specific investigation: ....

- Treatment Given:

Name of the Drug	*Dosag/Route/Frequency*	*Action*	*Side Effects*	*Nurses Responsibility*

Sl No.	*Needs Identified*	*Nursing Care Given*

- Antenatal advices: ....

....

....

....

....

General health condition of the mother: ....

Signature of the Student

Signature of the Supervisor

ANTENATAL EXAMINATION (3)

HISTORY COLLECTION

1. Baseline Data:

Name of the Mother: .... Date of Registration: ....

Age: .... Date of Admission: ....

Religion: .... Date of Assessment: ....

Hospital Number: .... Procedure Performed: ....

[Wards, Primary health center (PHC), Out patient department (OPD), Home]

Marital Status: ....

LMP: ....

EDD: ....

Period of gestation: ....

Obstetrical score:

G		P		L		A		S		D	

G-Gravida: .... P-Para: ....

L-Living: .... A-Abortion: ....

S-Still birth: .... D-Death: ....

Diagnosis: ....

Address: ....

2. Socioeconomic History:

Educational Status: .... Husband: ....

Wife: ....

Occupation: .... Husband: ....

Wife: ....

Total income: ....

Type of house: ....

Living standard:

Ownership of the house: Own house/Rented house

Lighting facility: ....

Environmental conditions of the house: Water facility: ....

Toilet facility: ....

Drainage, kitchen, garden: ....

Pet animals: ....

Cultural background: ....

3. Family History:

Sl No.	*Name of the Family Member*	*Age*	*Sex*	*Educational Status*	*Occupation*	*Relationship with the Mother*	*Health Status*
1.							
2.							
3.							
4.							
5.							
6.							

History of any

- Communicable diseases: ....
- Hereditary diseases: ....
- Twin pregnancy: ....
- Bad obstetrical history: ....

4. Personal History:
   - Dietary pattern: ....
   - Sleeping pattern: ....
   - Habits: ....
   - Bowel elimination: ....
   - Bladder elimination: ....
   - Immunization history: ....
   - Sexual history: ....
   - Drug history/Drug allergy: ....

5. Menstrual History: ....

....

6. Marital History: ....

....

7. Contraceptive History: ....

....

8. Previous Medical and Surgical History: ....

....

9. Previous Obstetrical History:

Sl No.	*Year*	*Antenatal Period*	*Intranatal Period*	*Postnatal Period*	*Alive/ Stillbirth*	*Sex*	*Weight*	*Remarks*
1								
2								
3								
4								
5								
6								

10. Present Obstetrical History:

a. Antenatal: ....

....

....

b. Intranatal: ....

....

....

c. Postnatal: ....

....

....

ANTENATAL EXAMINATION

1. General Examination:

General appearance: ....
Psychological status: ....
Head: ....
Hair: ....
Facial appearance: ....
Eyes: ....
Ears: ....
Nose: ....
Mouth: ....
Mucus membranes: ....
Gums: ....
Teeth: ....
Tongue: ....
Tonsils: ....
Neck: ....
Upper limbs: ....
Chest: ....
Lungs: ....
Heart: ....
Lower limbs: ....
Back: ....

Vital signs:

Temperature: ....
Pulse: ....
Respiration: ....
Blood pressure: ....

2. Obstetrical Examination:

a. Breast Examination:

Size and shape: ....
Sensation: ....
Primary areola: ....
Secondary areola: ....
Montgomery tubercles: ....
Colostrums: ....
Nipples: ....

b. Abdominal Examination:

Inspection: ....

Size of the abdomen: ....
Shape of the abdomen: ....

Contour of the abdominal wall:

- Skin changes on the abdomen: ....
- Previous operation scar: ....
- Striae gravidarum: ....
- Linea nigra: ....
- Umbilicus: Flattened/Protruded/Dimpled.

Visible fetal movement: ....

Flank region/Filled/Empty

Appearance of the skin infection: ....

Fundal Height (in cm): .... Abdominal girth (in cm): ....

- Abdominal palpation:

Fundal palpation: ....

Lateral palpation: ....

(i) Right lateral palpation: ....

(ii) Left lateral palpation: ....

Pelvic Palpation: ....

Pawlik's grip: ....

Auscultation: ....

- Findings:

Lie: .... Attitude: ....

Presentation: .... Position: ....

Denominator: ....

- Vaginal examination:

Discharge: ....

Sign of infection: .... Any other specify: ....

Investigation done:

Date	*Investigation Done*	*Mothers Value*	*Normal Value*	*Remarks*

Any other specific investigation: ....

- Treatment Given:

Name of the Drug	*Dosag/Route/Frequency*	*Action*	*Side Effects*	*Nurses Responsibility*

Sl No.	*Needs Identified*	*Nursing Care Given*

- Antenatal advices: ....
....
....
....
....

General health condition of the mother: ....

Signature of the Student

Signature of the Supervisor

ANTENATAL EXAMINATION (4)

HISTORY COLLECTION

1. Baseline Data:

   Name of the Mother: .... Date of Registration: ....

   Age: .... Date of Admission: ....

   Religion: .... Date of Assessment: ....

   Hospital Number: .... Procedure Performed: ....

   [Wards, Primary health center (PHC), Out patient department (OPD), Home]

   Marital Status: ....

   LMP: ....

   EDD: ....

   Period of gestation: ....

   Obstetrical score:

G		P		L		A		S		D	

   G-Gravida: .... P-Para: ....

   L-Living: .... A-Abortion: ....

   S-Still birth: .... D-Death: ....

   Diagnosis: ....

   Address: ....

2. Socioeconomic History:

   Educational Status: .... Husband: ....

   Wife: ....

   Occupation: .... Husband: ....

   Wife: ....

   Total income: ....

   Type of house: ....

   Living standard:

   Ownership of the house: Own house/Rented house

   Lighting facility: ....

   Environmental conditions of the house: Water facility: ....

   Toilet facility: ....

Drainage, kitchen, garden: ....

Pet animals: ....

Cultural background: ....

3. Family History:

Sl No.	*Name of the Family Member*	*Age*	*Sex*	*Educational Status*	*Occupation*	*Relationship with the Mother*	*Health Status*
1.							
2.							
3.							
4.							
5.							
6.							

History of any

- Communicable diseases: ....
- Hereditary diseases: ....
- Twin pregnancy: ....
- Bad obstetrical history: ....

4. Personal History:

- Dietary pattern: ....
- Sleeping pattern: ....
- Habits: ....
- Bowel elimination: ....
- Bladder elimination: ....
- Immunization history: ....
- Sexual history: ....
- Drug history/Drug allergy: ....

5. Menstrual History: ....

....

6. Marital History: ....

....

7. Contraceptive History: ....

....

8. Previous Medical and Surgical History: ....

....

9. Previous Obstetrical History:

Sl No.	*Year*	*Antenatal Period*	*Intranatal Period*	*Postnatal Period*	*Alive/ Stillbirth*	*Sex*	*Weight*	*Remarks*
1								
2								
3								
4								
5								
6								

10. Present Obstetrical History:

    a. Antenatal: ....

    ....

    ....

    b. Intranatal: ....

    ....

    ....

    c. Postnatal: ....

    ....

    ....

ANTENATAL EXAMINATION

1. General Examination:

General appearance: .... Psychological status: ....

Head: .... Hair: ....

Facial appearance: .... Eyes: ....

Ears: .... Nose: ....

Mouth: .... Mucus membranes: ....

Gums: .... Teeth: ....

Tongue: .... Tonsils: ....

Neck: .... Upper limbs: ....

Chest: .... Lungs: ....

Heart: .... Lower limbs: ....

Back: ....

Vital signs:

Temperature: .... Pulse: ....

Respiration: .... Blood pressure: ....

2. Obstetrical Examination:

a. Breast Examination:

Size and shape: .... Sensation: ....

Primary areola: .... Secondary areola: ....

Montgomery tubercles: .... Colostrums: ....

Nipples: ....

b. Abdominal Examination:

Inspection: ....

Size of the abdomen: .... Shape of the abdomen: ....

Contour of the abdominal wall:

- Skin changes on the abdomen: ....
- Previous operation scar: ....
- Striae gravidarum: ....
- Linea nigra: ....
- Umbilicus: Flattened/Protruded/Dimpled.

Visible fetal movement: ....

Flank region/Filled/Empty

Appearance of the skin infection: ....

Fundal Height (in cm): .... Abdominal girth (in cm): ....

- Abdominal palpation:

Fundal palpation: ....

Lateral palpation: ....

(i) Right lateral palpation: ....

(ii) Left lateral palpation: ....

Pelvic Palpation: ....

Pawlik's grip: ....

Auscultation: ....

- Findings:

Lie: .... Attitude: ....

Presentation: .... Position: ....

Denominator: ....

- Vaginal examination:

Discharge: ....

Sign of infection: .... Any other specify: ....

Investigation done:

Date	*Investigation Done*	*Mothers Value*	*Normal Value*	*Remarks*

Any other specific investigation: ....

- Treatment Given:

Name of the Drug	*Dosag/Route/Frequency*	*Action*	*Side Effects*	*Nurses Responsibility*

Sl No.	*Needs Identified*	*Nursing Care Given*

- Antenatal advices: ....
....
....
....
....

General health condition of the mother: ....

Signature of the Student

Signature of the Supervisor

ANTENATAL EXAMINATION (5)

HISTORY COLLECTION

1. Baseline Data:

Name of the Mother: ....

Date of Registration: ....

Age: ....

Date of Admission: ....

Religion: ....

Date of Assessment: ....

Hospital Number: ....

Procedure Performed: ....

[Wards, Primary health center (PHC), Out patient department (OPD), Home]

Marital Status: ....

LMP: ....

EDD: ....

Period of gestation: ....

Obstetrical score:

G		P		L		A		S		D	

G-Gravida: ....

P-Para: ....

L-Living: ....

A-Abortion: ....

S-Still birth: ....

D-Death: ....

Diagnosis: ....

Address: ....

2. Socioeconomic History:

Educational Status: ....

Husband: ....

Wife: ....

Occupation: ....

Husband: ....

Wife: ....

Total income: ....

Type of house: ....

Living standard:

Ownership of the house: Own house/Rented house

Lighting facility: ....

Environmental conditions of the house:

Water facility: ....

Toilet facility: ....

Drainage, kitchen, garden: ....

Pet animals: ....

Cultural background: ....

3. Family History:

Sl No.	*Name of the Family Member*	*Age*	*Sex*	*Educational Status*	*Occupation*	*Relationship with the Mother*	*Health Status*
1.							
2.							
3.							
4.							
5.							
6.							

History of any

- Communicable diseases: ....
- Hereditary diseases: ....
- Twin pregnancy: ....
- Bad obstetrical history: ....

4. Personal History:
   - Dietary pattern: ....
   - Sleeping pattern: ....
   - Habits: ....
   - Bowel elimination: ....
   - Bladder elimination: ....
   - Immunization history: ....
   - Sexual history: ....
   - Drug history/Drug allergy: ....

5. Menstrual History: ....

....

6. Marital History: ....

....

7. Contraceptive History: ....

....

8. Previous Medical and Surgical History: ....

....

9. Previous Obstetrical History:

Sl No.	*Year*	*Antenatal Period*	*Intranatal Period*	*Postnatal Period*	*Alive/ Stillbirth*	*Sex*	*Weight*	*Remarks*
1								
2								
3								
4								
5								
6								

10. Present Obstetrical History:

a. Antenatal: ....

....

....

b. Intranatal: ....

....

....

c. Postnatal: ....

....

....

ANTENATAL EXAMINATION

1. General Examination:

General appearance: ....

Psychological status: ....

Head: ....

Hair: ....

Facial appearance: ....

Eyes: ....

Ears: ....

Nose: ....

Mouth: ....

Mucus membranes: ....

Gums: ....

Teeth: ....

Tongue: ....

Tonsils: ....

Neck: ....

Upper limbs: ....

Chest: ....

Lungs: ....

Heart: ....

Lower limbs: ....

Back: ....

Vital signs:

Temperature: ....

Pulse: ....

Respiration: ....

Blood pressure: ....

2. Obstetrical Examination:

   a. Breast Examination:

   Size and shape: ....

   Sensation: ....

   Primary areola: ....

   Secondary areola: ....

   Montgomery tubercles: ....

   Colostrums: ....

   Nipples: ....

   b. Abdominal Examination:

   Inspection: ....

   Size of the abdomen: ....

   Shape of the abdomen: ....

   Contour of the abdominal wall:

   - Skin changes on the abdomen: ....
   - Previous operation scar: ....
   - Striae gravidarum: ....
   - Linea nigra: ....
   - Umbilicus: Flattened/Protruded/Dimpled.

     Visible fetal movement: ....

     Flank region/Filled/Empty

Appearance of the skin infection: ....

Fundal Height (in cm): .... Abdominal girth (in cm): ....

- Abdominal palpation:

  Fundal palpation: ....

  Lateral palpation: ....

  (i) Right lateral palpation: ....

  (ii) Left lateral palpation: ....

  Pelvic Palpation: ....

  Pawlik's grip: ....

  Auscultation: ....

- Findings:

  Lie: .... Attitude: ....

  Presentation: .... Position: ....

  Denominator: ....

- Vaginal examination:

  Discharge: ....

  Sign of infection: .... Any other specify: ....

  Investigation done:

Date	*Investigation Done*	*Mothers Value*	*Normal Value*	*Remarks*

Any other specific investigation: ....

- Treatment Given:

Name of the Drug	*Dosag/Route/Frequency*	*Action*	*Side Effects*	*Nurses Responsibility*

Sl No.	*Needs Identified*	*Nursing Care Given*

- Antenatal advices: ....
....
....
....
....

General health condition of the mother: ....

Signature of the Student

Signature of the Supervisor

ANTENATAL EXAMINATION (6)

HISTORY COLLECTION

1. Baseline Data:

Name of the Mother: ....

Date of Registration: ....

Age: ....

Date of Admission: ....

Religion: ....

Date of Assessment: ....

Hospital Number: ....

Procedure Performed: ....

[Wards, Primary health center (PHC), Out patient department (OPD), Home]

Marital Status: ....

LMP: ....

EDD: ....

Period of gestation: ....

Obstetrical score:

G		P		L		A		S		D	

G-Gravida: ....

P-Para: ....

L-Living: ....

A-Abortion: ....

S-Still birth: ....

D-Death: ....

Diagnosis: ....

Address: ....

2. Socioeconomic History:

Educational Status: ....

Husband: ....

Wife: ....

Occupation: ....

Husband: ....

Wife: ....

Total income: ....

Type of house: ....

Living standard:

Ownership of the house: Own house/Rented house

Lighting facility: ....

Environmental conditions of the house:

Water facility: ....

Toilet facility: ....

Drainage, kitchen, garden: ....

Pet animals: ....

Cultural background: ....

3. Family History:

Sl No.	*Name of the Family Member*	*Age*	*Sex*	*Educational Status*	*Occupation*	*Relationship with the Mother*	*Health Status*
1.							
2.							
3.							
4.							
5.							
6.							

History of any

- Communicable diseases: ....
- Hereditary diseases: ....
- Twin pregnancy: ....
- Bad obstetrical history: ....

4. Personal History:

- Dietary pattern: ....
- Sleeping pattern: ....
- Habits: ....
- Bowel elimination: ....
- Bladder elimination: ....
- Immunization history: ....
- Sexual history: ....
- Drug history/Drug allergy: ....

5. Menstrual History: ....

....

6. Marital History: ....

....

7. Contraceptive History: ....

....

8. Previous Medical and Surgical History: ....

....

9. Previous Obstetrical History:

Sl No.	*Year*	*Antenatal Period*	*Intranatal Period*	*Postnatal Period*	*Alive/ Stillbirth*	*Sex*	*Weight*	*Remarks*
1								
2								
3								
4								
5								
6								

10. Present Obstetrical History:

    a. Antenatal: ....

    ....

    ....

    b. Intranatal: ....

    ....

    ....

    c. Postnatal: ....

    ....

    ....

ANTENATAL EXAMINATION

1. General Examination:

General appearance: .... Psychological status: ....

Head: .... Hair: ....

Facial appearance: .... Eyes: ....

Ears: .... Nose: ....

Mouth: .... Mucus membranes: ....

Gums: .... Teeth: ....

Tongue: .... Tonsils: ....

Neck: .... Upper limbs: ....

Chest: .... Lungs: ....

Heart: .... Lower limbs: ....

Back: ....

Vital signs:

Temperature: .... Pulse: ....

Respiration: .... Blood pressure: ....

2. Obstetrical Examination:

   a. Breast Examination:

   Size and shape: .... Sensation: ....

   Primary areola: .... Secondary areola: ....

   Montgomery tubercles: .... Colostrums: ....

   Nipples: ....

   b. Abdominal Examination:

   Inspection: ....

   Size of the abdomen: .... Shape of the abdomen: ....

   Contour of the abdominal wall:

   - Skin changes on the abdomen: ....
   - Previous operation scar: ....
   - Striae gravidarum: ....
   - Linea nigra: ....
   - Umbilicus: Flattened/Protruded/Dimpled.

     Visible fetal movement: ....

     Flank region/Filled/Empty

Appearance of the skin infection: ....

Fundal Height (in cm): .... Abdominal girth (in cm): ....

- Abdominal palpation:

Fundal palpation: ....

Lateral palpation: ....

(i) Right lateral palpation: ....

(ii) Left lateral palpation: ....

Pelvic Palpation: ....

Pawlik's grip: ....

Auscultation: ....

- Findings:

Lie: .... Attitude: ....

Presentation: .... Position: ....

Denominator: ....

- Vaginal examination:

Discharge: ....

Sign of infection: .... Any other specify: ....

Investigation done:

Date	*Investigation Done*	*Mothers Value*	*Normal Value*	*Remarks*

Any other specific investigation: ....

- Treatment Given:

Name of the Drug	*Dosag/Route/Frequency*	*Action*	*Side Effects*	*Nurses Responsibility*

Sl No.	*Needs Identified*	*Nursing Care Given*

- Antenatal advices: ....
....
....
....
....

General health condition of the mother: ....

Signature of the Student

Signature of the Supervisor

ANTENATAL EXAMINATION (7)

HISTORY COLLECTION

1. Baseline Data:

Name of the Mother: .... Date of Registration: ....

Age: .... Date of Admission: ....

Religion: .... Date of Assessment: ....

Hospital Number: .... Procedure Performed: ....

[Wards, Primary health center (PHC), Out patient department (OPD), Home]

Marital Status: ....

LMP: ....

EDD: ....

Period of gestation: ....

Obstetrical score:

G		P		L		A		S		D	

G-Gravida: .... P-Para: ....

L-Living: .... A-Abortion: ....

S-Still birth: .... D-Death: ....

Diagnosis: ....

Address: ....

2. Socioeconomic History:

Educational Status: .... Husband: ....

Wife: ....

Occupation: .... Husband: ....

Wife: ....

Total income: ....

Type of house: ....

Living standard:

Ownership of the house: Own house/Rented house

Lighting facility: ....

Environmental conditions of the house: Water facility: ....

Toilet facility: ....

Drainage, kitchen, garden: ....

Pet animals: ....

Cultural background: ....

3. Family History:

Sl No.	*Name of the Family Member*	*Age*	*Sex*	*Educational Status*	*Occupation*	*Relationship with the Mother*	*Health Status*
1.							
2.							
3.							
4.							
5.							
6.							

History of any

- Communicable diseases: ....
- Hereditary diseases: ....
- Twin pregnancy: ....
- Bad obstetrical history: ....

4. Personal History:
   - Dietary pattern: ....
   - Sleeping pattern: ....
   - Habits: ....
   - Bowel elimination: ....
   - Bladder elimination: ....
   - Immunization history: ....
   - Sexual history: ....
   - Drug history/Drug allergy: ....

5. Menstrual History: ....

....

6. Marital History: ....

....

7. Contraceptive History: ....

....

8. Previous Medical and Surgical History: ....

....

9. Previous Obstetrical History:

Sl No.	*Year*	*Antenatal Period*	*Intranatal Period*	*Postnatal Period*	*Alive/ Stillbirth*	*Sex*	*Weight*	*Remarks*
1								
2								
3								
4								
5								
6								

10. Present Obstetrical History:

a. Antenatal: ....

....

....

b. Intranatal: ....

....

....

c. Postnatal: ....

....

....

ANTENATAL EXAMINATION

1. General Examination:

General appearance: .... Psychological status: ....

Head: .... Hair: ....

Facial appearance: .... Eyes: ....

Ears: .... Nose: ....

Mouth: .... Mucus membranes: ....

Gums: .... Teeth: ....

Tongue: .... Tonsils: ....

Neck: .... Upper limbs: ....

Chest: .... Lungs: ....

Heart: .... Lower limbs: ....

Back: ....

Vital signs:

Temperature: .... Pulse: ....

Respiration: .... Blood pressure: ....

2. Obstetrical Examination:

a. Breast Examination:

Size and shape: .... Sensation: ....

Primary areola: .... Secondary areola: ....

Montgomery tubercles: .... Colostrums: ....

Nipples: ....

b. Abdominal Examination:

Inspection: ....

Size of the abdomen: .... Shape of the abdomen: ....

Contour of the abdominal wall:

- Skin changes on the abdomen: ....
- Previous operation scar: ....
- Striae gravidarum: ....
- Linea nigra: ....
- Umbilicus: Flattened/Protruded/Dimpled.

Visible fetal movement: ....

Flank region/Filled/Empty

Appearance of the skin infection: ....

Fundal Height (in cm): .... Abdominal girth (in cm): ....

- Abdominal palpation:

Fundal palpation: ....

Lateral palpation: ....

(i) Right lateral palpation: ....

(ii) Left lateral palpation: ....

Pelvic Palpation: ....

Pawlik's grip: ....

Auscultation: ....

- Findings:

Lie: .... Attitude: ....

Presentation: .... Position: ....

Denominator: ....

- Vaginal examination:

Discharge: ....

Sign of infection: .... Any other specify: ....

Investigation done:

Date	*Investigation Done*	*Mothers Value*	*Normal Value*	*Remarks*

Any other specific investigation: ....

- Treatment Given:

Name of the Drug	*Dosag/Route/Frequency*	*Action*	*Side Effects*	*Nurses Responsibility*

Sl No.	*Needs Identified*	*Nursing Care Given*

- Antenatal advices: ....

....

....

....

....

General health condition of the mother: ....

Signature of the Student

Signature of the Supervisor

ANTENATAL EXAMINATION (8)

HISTORY COLLECTION

1. Baseline Data:

Name of the Mother: .... Date of Registration: ....

Age: .... Date of Admission: ....

Religion: .... Date of Assessment: ....

Hospital Number: .... Procedure Performed: ....

[Wards, Primary health center (PHC), Out patient department (OPD), Home]

Marital Status: ....

LMP: ....

EDD: ....

Period of gestation: ....

Obstetrical score:

G		P		L		A		S		D	

G-Gravida: .... P-Para: ....

L-Living: .... A-Abortion: ....

S-Still birth: .... D-Death: ....

Diagnosis: ....

Address: ....

2. Socioeconomic History:

Educational Status: .... Husband: ....

Wife: ....

Occupation: .... Husband: ....

Wife: ....

Total income: ....

Type of house: ....

Living standard:

Ownership of the house: Own house/Rented house

Lighting facility: ....

Environmental conditions of the house: Water facility: ....

Toilet facility: ....

Drainage, kitchen, garden: ....

Pet animals: ....

Cultural background: ....

3. Family History:

Sl No.	Name of the Family Member	Age	Sex	Educational Status	Occupation	Relationship with the Mother	Health Status
1.							
2.							
3.							
4.							
5.							
6.							

History of any

- Communicable diseases: ....
- Hereditary diseases: ....
- Twin pregnancy: ....
- Bad obstetrical history: ....

4. Personal History:

- Dietary pattern: ....
- Sleeping pattern: ....
- Habits: ....
- Bowel elimination: ....
- Bladder elimination: ....
- Immunization history: ....
- Sexual history: ....
- Drug history/Drug allergy: ....

5. Menstrual History: ....

....

6. Marital History: ....

....

7. Contraceptive History: ....

....

8. Previous Medical and Surgical History: ....

....

9. Previous Obstetrical History:

Sl No.	*Year*	*Antenatal Period*	*Intranatal Period*	*Postnatal Period*	*Alive/ Stillbirth*	*Sex*	*Weight*	*Remarks*
1								
2								
3								
4								
5								
6								

10. Present Obstetrical History:

   a. Antenatal: ....

   ....

   ....

   b. Intranatal: ....

   ....

   ....

   c. Postnatal: ....

   ....

   ....

ANTENATAL EXAMINATION

1. General Examination:

General appearance: .... Psychological status: ....

Head: .... Hair: ....

Facial appearance: .... Eyes: ....

Ears: .... Nose: ....

Mouth: .... Mucus membranes: ....

Gums: .... Teeth: ....

Tongue: .... Tonsils: ....

Neck: .... Upper limbs: ....

Chest: .... Lungs: ....

Heart: .... Lower limbs: ....

Back: ....

Vital signs:

Temperature: .... Pulse: ....

Respiration: .... Blood pressure: ....

2. Obstetrical Examination:

a. Breast Examination:

Size and shape: .... Sensation: ....

Primary areola: .... Secondary areola: ....

Montgomery tubercles: .... Colostrums: ....

Nipples: ....

b. Abdominal Examination:

Inspection: ....

Size of the abdomen: .... Shape of the abdomen: ....

Contour of the abdominal wall:

- Skin changes on the abdomen: ....
- Previous operation scar: ....
- Striae gravidarum: ....
- Linea nigra: ....
- Umbilicus: Flattened/Protruded/Dimpled.

Visible fetal movement: ....

Flank region/Filled/Empty

Appearance of the skin infection: ....

Fundal Height (in cm): .... Abdominal girth (in cm): ....

- Abdominal palpation:

Fundal palpation: ....

Lateral palpation: ....

(i) Right lateral palpation: ....

(ii) Left lateral palpation: ....

Pelvic Palpation: ....

Pawlik's grip: ....

Auscultation: ....

- Findings:

Lie: .... Attitude: ....

Presentation: .... Position: ....

Denominator: ....

- Vaginal examination:

Discharge: ....

Sign of infection: .... Any other specify: ....

Investigation done:

Date	*Investigation Done*	*Mothers Value*	*Normal Value*	*Remarks*

Any other specific investigation: ....

- Treatment Given:

Name of the Drug	*Dosag/Route/Frequency*	*Action*	*Side Effects*	*Nurses Responsibility*

Sl No.	*Needs Identified*	*Nursing Care Given*

- Antenatal advices: ....

....

....

....

....

General health condition of the mother: ....

Signature of the Student

Signature of the Supervisor

ANTENATAL EXAMINATION (9)

HISTORY COLLECTION

1. Baseline Data:

Name of the Mother: .... Date of Registration: ....

Age: .... Date of Admission: ....

Religion: .... Date of Assessment: ....

Hospital Number: .... Procedure Performed: ....

[Wards, Primary health center (PHC), Out patient department (OPD), Home]

Marital Status: ....

LMP: ....

EDD: ....

Period of gestation: ....

Obstetrical score:

G		P		L		A		S		D	

G-Gravida: .... P-Para: ....

L-Living: .... A-Abortion: ....

S-Still birth: .... D-Death: ....

Diagnosis: ....

Address: ....

2. Socioeconomic History:

Educational Status: .... Husband: ....

Wife: ....

Occupation: .... Husband: ....

Wife: ....

Total income: ....

Type of house: ....

Living standard:

Ownership of the house: Own house/Rented house

Lighting facility: ....

Environmental conditions of the house: Water facility: ....

Toilet facility: ....

Drainage, kitchen, garden: ....

Pet animals: ....

Cultural background: ....

3. Family History:

Sl No.	Name of the Family Member	Age	Sex	Educational Status	Occupation	Relationship with the Mother	Health Status
1.							
2.							
3.							
4.							
5.							
6.							

History of any

- Communicable diseases: ....
- Hereditary diseases: ....
- Twin pregnancy: ....
- Bad obstetrical history: ....

4. Personal History:
   - Dietary pattern: ....
   - Sleeping pattern: ....
   - Habits: ....
   - Bowel elimination: ....
   - Bladder elimination: ....
   - Immunization history: ....
   - Sexual history: ....
   - Drug history/Drug allergy: ....

5. Menstrual History: ....

....

6. Marital History: ....

....

7. Contraceptive History: ....

....

8. Previous Medical and Surgical History: ....

....

9. Previous Obstetrical History:

Sl No.	*Year*	*Antenatal Period*	*Intranatal Period*	*Postnatal Period*	*Alive/ Stillbirth*	*Sex*	*Weight*	*Remarks*
1								
2								
3								
4								
5								
6								

10. Present Obstetrical History:

 a. Antenatal: ....

 ....

 ....

 b. Intranatal: ....

 ....

 ....

 c. Postnatal: ....

 ....

 ....

ANTENATAL EXAMINATION

1. General Examination:

General appearance: ....

Psychological status: ....

Head: ....

Hair: ....

Facial appearance: ....

Eyes: ....

Ears: ....

Nose: ....

Mouth: ....

Mucus membranes: ....

Gums: ....

Teeth: ....

Tongue: ....

Tonsils: ....

Neck: ....

Upper limbs: ....

Chest: ....

Lungs: ....

Heart: ....

Lower limbs: ....

Back: ....

Vital signs:

Temperature: ....

Pulse: ....

Respiration: ....

Blood pressure: ....

2. Obstetrical Examination:

a. Breast Examination:

Size and shape: ....

Sensation: ....

Primary areola: ....

Secondary areola: ....

Montgomery tubercles: ....

Colostrums: ....

Nipples: ....

b. Abdominal Examination:

Inspection: ....

Size of the abdomen: ....

Shape of the abdomen: ....

Contour of the abdominal wall: ....

- Skin changes on the abdomen: ....
- Previous operation scar: ....
- Striae gravidarum: ....
- Linea nigra: ....
- Umbilicus: Flattened/Protruded/Dimpled.

Visible fetal movement: ....

Flank region/Filled/Empty

Appearance of the skin infection: ....

Fundal Height (in cm): .... Abdominal girth (in cm): ....

- Abdominal palpation:

Fundal palpation: ....

Lateral palpation: ....

(i) Right lateral palpation: ....

(ii) Left lateral palpation: ....

Pelvic Palpation: ....

Pawlik's grip: ....

Auscultation: ....

- Findings:

Lie: .... Attitude: ....

Presentation: .... Position: ....

Denominator: ....

- Vaginal examination:

Discharge: ....

Sign of infection: .... Any other specify: ....

Investigation done:

Date	*Investigation Done*	*Mothers Value*	*Normal Value*	*Remarks*

Any other specific investigation: ....

- Treatment Given:

Name of the Drug	*Dosag/Route/Frequency*	*Action*	*Side Effects*	*Nurses Responsibility*

Sl No.	*Needs Identified*	*Nursing Care Given*

- Antenatal advices: ....
....
....
....
....

General health condition of the mother: ....

Signature of the Student

Signature of the Supervisor

ANTENATAL EXAMINATION (10)

HISTORY COLLECTION

1. Baseline Data:

Name of the Mother: ....

Date of Registration: ....

Age: ....

Date of Admission: ....

Religion: ....

Date of Assessment: ....

Hospital Number: ....

Procedure Performed: ....

[Wards, Primary health center (PHC), Out patient department (OPD), Home]

Marital Status: ....

LMP: ....

EDD: ....

Period of gestation: ....

Obstetrical score:

G		P		L		A		S		D	

G-Gravida: ....

P-Para: ....

L-Living: ....

A-Abortion: ....

S-Still birth: ....

D-Death: ....

Diagnosis: ....

Address: ....

2. Socioeconomic History:

Educational Status: ....

Husband: ....

Wife: ....

Occupation: ....

Husband: ....

Wife: ....

Total income: ....

Type of house: ....

Living standard:

Ownership of the house: Own house/Rented house

Lighting facility: ....

Environmental conditions of the house:

Water facility: ....

Toilet facility: ....

Drainage, kitchen, garden: ....

Pet animals: ....

Cultural background: ....

3. Family History:

Sl No.	*Name of the Family Member*	*Age*	*Sex*	*Educational Status*	*Occupation*	*Relationship with the Mother*	*Health Status*
1.							
2.							
3.							
4.							
5.							
6.							

History of any

- Communicable diseases: ....
- Hereditary diseases: ....
- Twin pregnancy: ....
- Bad obstetrical history: ....

4. Personal History:
   - Dietary pattern: ....
   - Sleeping pattern: ....
   - Habits: ....
   - Bowel elimination: ....
   - Bladder elimination: ....
   - Immunization history: ....
   - Sexual history: ....
   - Drug history/Drug allergy: ....

5. Menstrual History: ....

....

6. Marital History: ....

....

7. Contraceptive History: ....

....

8. Previous Medical and Surgical History: ....

....

9. Previous Obstetrical History:

Sl No.	*Year*	*Antenatal Period*	*Intranatal Period*	*Postnatal Period*	*Alive/ Stillbirth*	*Sex*	*Weight*	*Remarks*
1								
2								
3								
4								
5								
6								

10. Present Obstetrical History:

a. Antenatal: ....

....

....

b. Intranatal: ....

....

....

c. Postnatal: ....

....

....

ANTENATAL EXAMINATION

1. General Examination:

General appearance: ....

Psychological status: ....

Head: ....

Hair: ....

Facial appearance: ....

Eyes: ....

Ears: ....

Nose: ....

Mouth: ....

Mucus membranes: ....

Gums: ....

Teeth: ....

Tongue: ....

Tonsils: ....

Neck: ....

Upper limbs: ....

Chest: ....

Lungs: ....

Heart: ....

Lower limbs: ....

Back: ....

Vital signs:

Temperature: ....

Pulse: ....

Respiration: ....

Blood pressure: ....

2. Obstetrical Examination:

   a. Breast Examination:

   Size and shape: ....

   Sensation: ....

   Primary areola: ....

   Secondary areola: ....

   Montgomery tubercles: ....

   Colostrums: ....

   Nipples: ....

   b. Abdominal Examination:

   Inspection: ....

   Size of the abdomen: ....

   Shape of the abdomen: ....

   Contour of the abdominal wall: ....

   - Skin changes on the abdomen: ....
   - Previous operation scar: ....
   - Striae gravidarum: ....
   - Linea nigra: ....
   - Umbilicus: Flattened/Protruded/Dimpled.

     Visible fetal movement: ....

     Flank region/Filled/Empty

Appearance of the skin infection: ....

Fundal Height (in cm): .... Abdominal girth (in cm): ....

- Abdominal palpation:

Fundal palpation: ....

Lateral palpation: ....

(i) Right lateral palpation: ....

(ii) Left lateral palpation: ....

Pelvic Palpation: ....

Pawlik's grip: ....

Auscultation: ....

- Findings:

Lie: .... Attitude: ....

Presentation: .... Position: ....

Denominator: ....

- Vaginal examination:

Discharge: ....

Sign of infection: .... Any other specify: ....

Investigation done:

Date	*Investigation Done*	*Mothers Value*	*Normal Value*	*Remarks*

Any other specific investigation: ....

- Treatment Given:

Name of the Drug	*Dosag/Route/Frequency*	*Action*	*Side Effects*	*Nurses Responsibility*

Sl No.	*Needs Identified*	*Nursing Care Given*

- Antenatal advices: ....
....
....
....
....

General health condition of the mother: ....

Signature of the Student

Signature of the Supervisor

CHAPTER 2

Antenatal Examination and Care (Normal and High-risk Mother)

ANTENATAL EXAMINATION AND CARE

(Including High-risk Mothers)

Sl No.	*Register No.*	*Name of the Mother*	*Age*	*Date of Examination*	*Obstetrical Score*	*LMP*	*EDD*	*Gestational Age (week)*	*Fundal Height (in cm)*	*Abdominal Girth (in cm)*	*Findings*	*FHS*	*General Condition of the Mother*						*Other investigations and findings*	*Treatment and Advice Given*
													Weight (kg)	*Height of the Mother*	*Blood Group*	*BP (mm Hg)*	*Urine*			
																	Albumin	*Sugar*		
1.																				
2.																				
3.																				
4.																				
5.																				
6.																				
7.																				
8.																				
9.																				
10.																				

ANTENATAL EXAMINATION (1)

HISTORY COLLECTION

1. Baseline Data:

Name of the Mother: .... Date of Registration: ....

Age: .... Date of Admission: ....

Religion: .... Date of Assessment: ....

Hospital Number: .... Procedure Performed: ....

[Wards, Primary health center (PHC), Out patient department (OPD), Home]

Marital Status: ....

LMP: ....

EDD: ....

Period of gestation: ....

Obstetrical score:

G		P		L		A		S		D	

G-Gravida: .... P-Para: ....

L-Living: .... A-Abortion: ....

S-Still birth: .... D-Death: ....

Diagnosis: ....

Address: ....

2. Socioeconomic History:

Educational Status: .... Husband: ....

Wife: ....

Occupation: .... Husband: ....

Wife: ....

Total income: ....

Type of house: ....

Living standard:

Ownership of the house: Own house/Rented house

Lighting facility: ....

Environmental conditions of the house: Water facility: ....

Toilet facility: ....

Drainage, kitchen, garden: ....

Pet animals: ....

Cultural background: ....

3. Family History:

Sl No.	*Name of the Family Member*	*Age*	*Sex*	*Educational Status*	*Occupation*	*Relationship with the Mother*	*Health Status*
1.							
2.							
3.							
4.							
5.							
6.							

History of any

- Communicable diseases: ....
- Hereditary diseases: ....
- Twin pregnancy: ....
- Bad obstetrical history: ....

4. Personal History:
   - Dietary pattern: ....
   - Sleeping pattern: ....
   - Habits: ....
   - Bowel elimination: ....
   - Bladder elimination: ....
   - Immunization history: ....
   - Sexual history: ....
   - Drug history/Drug allergy: ....

5. Menstrual History: ....

....

6. Marital History: ....

....

7. Contraceptive History: ....

....

8. Previous Medical and Surgical History: ....

....

9. Previous Obstetrical History:

Sl No.	*Year*	*Antenatal Period*	*Intranatal Period*	*Postnatal Period*	*Alive/ Stillbirth*	*Sex*	*Weight*	*Remarks*
1								
2								
3								
4								
5								
6								

10. Present Obstetrical History:

    a. Antenatal: ....

    ....

    ....

    b. Intranatal: ....

    ....

    ....

    c. Postnatal: ....

    ....

    ....

ANTENATAL EXAMINATION

1. General Examination:

General appearance: ....

Psychological status: ....

Head: ....

Hair: ....

Facial appearance: ....

Eyes: ....

Ears: ....

Nose: ....

Mouth: ....

Mucus membranes: ....

Gums: ....

Teeth: ....

Tongue: ....

Tonsils: ....

Neck: ....

Upper limbs: ....

Chest: ....

Lungs: ....

Heart: ....

Lower limbs: ....

Back: ....

Vital signs: ....

Temperature: ....

Pulse: ....

Respiration: ....

Blood pressure: ....

2. Obstetrical Examination:

a. Breast Examination:

Size and shape: ....

Sensation: ....

Primary areola: ....

Secondary areola: ....

Montgomery tubercles: ....

Colostrums: ....

Nipples: ....

b. Abdominal Examination:

Inspection: ....

Size of the abdomen: ....

Shape of the abdomen: ....

Contour of the abdominal wall:

- Skin changes on the abdomen: ....
- Previous operation scar: ....
- Striae gravidarum: ....
- Linea nigra: ....
- Umbilicus: Flattened/Protruded/Dimpled.

Visible fetal movement: ....

Flank region/Filled/Empty

Appearance of the skin infection: ....

Fundal Height (in cm): .... Abdominal girth (in cm): ....

- Abdominal palpation:

Fundal palpation: ....

Lateral palpation: ....

(i) Right lateral palpation: ....

(ii) Left lateral palpation: ....

Pelvic Palpation: ....

Pawlik's grip: ....

Auscultation: ....

- Findings:

Lie: .... Attitude: ....

Presentation: .... Position: ....

Denominator: ....

- Vaginal examination:

Discharge: .... Normal: ....

Abnormal: .... Foul smelling: ....

(VDRL) infection: ....

Investigation done

Date	*Investigation Done*	*Mothers Value*	*Normal Value*	*Remarks*

Any other specific investigation: ....

- Treatment Given: ....

....

....

....

....

Name of the Drug	*Dosag/Route/Frequency*	*Action*	*Side Effects*	*Nurses Responsibility*

Sl No.	*Needs Identified*	*Nursing Care Given*

- Antenatal advices: ....

General health condition of the mother: ....

Signature of the Student

Signature of the Supervisor

NURSING CARE PLAN

Assessment	*Nursing Diagnosis*	*Goals*	*Nursing Intervention*	*Rationale*	*Nursing Implementation*	*Evaluation*

NURSING CARE PLAN

Assessment	*Nursing Diagnosis*	*Goals*	*Nursing Intervention*	*Rationale*	*Nursing Implementation*	*Evaluation*

NURSING CARE PLAN

Assessment	*Nursing Diagnosis*	*Goals*	*Nursing Intervention*	*Rationale*	*Nursing Implementation*	*Evaluation*

ANTENATAL EXAMINATION (2)

HISTORY COLLECTION

1. Baseline Data:

Name of the Mother: .... Date of Registration: ....

Age: .... Date of Admission: ....

Religion: .... Date of Assessment: ....

Hospital Number: .... Procedure Performed: ....

[Wards, Primary health center (PHC), Out patient department (OPD), Home]

Marital Status: ....

LMP: ....

EDD: ....

Period of gestation: ....

Obstetrical score:

G		P		L		A		S		D	

G-Gravida: .... P-Para: ....

L-Living: .... A-Abortion: ....

S-Still birth: .... D-Death: ....

Diagnosis: ....

Address: ....

2. Socioeconomic History:

Educational Status: .... Husband: ....

Wife: ....

Occupation: .... Husband: ....

Wife: ....

Total income: ....

Type of house: ....

Living standard:

Ownership of the house: Own house/Rented house

Lighting facility: ....

Environmental conditions of the house: Water facility: ....

Toilet facility: ....

Drainage, kitchen, garden: ....

Pet animals: ....

Cultural background: ....

3. Family History:

Sl No.	*Name of the Family Member*	*Age*	*Sex*	*Educational Status*	*Occupation*	*Relationship with the Mother*	*Health Status*
1.							
2.							
3.							
4.							
5.							
6.							

History of any

- Communicable diseases: ....
- Hereditary diseases: ....
- Twin pregnancy: ....
- Bad obstetrical history: ....

4. Personal History:

- Dietary pattern: ....
- Sleeping pattern: ....
- Habits: ....
- Bowel elimination: ....
- Bladder elimination: ....
- Immunization history: ....
- Sexual history: ....
- Drug history/Drug allergy: ....

5. Menstrual History: ....

....

6. Marital History: ....

....

7. Contraceptive History: ....

....

8. Previous Medical and Surgical History: ....

....

9. Previous Obstetrical History:

Sl No.	*Year*	*Antenatal Period*	*Intranatal Period*	*Postnatal Period*	*Alive/ Stillbirth*	*Sex*	*Weight*	*Remarks*
1								
2								
3								
4								
5								
6								

10. Present Obstetrical History:

    a. Antenatal: ....

    ....

    ....

    b. Intranatal: ....

    ....

    ....

    c. Postnatal: ....

    ....

    ....

ANTENATAL EXAMINATION

1. General Examination:

General appearance: .... Psychological status: ....

Head: .... Hair: ....

Facial appearance: .... Eyes: ....

Ears: .... Nose: ....

Mouth: .... Mucus membranes: ....

Gums: .... Teeth: ....

Tongue: .... Tonsils: ....

Neck: .... Upper limbs: ....

Chest: .... Lungs: ....

Heart: .... Lower limbs: ....

Back: .... Vital signs: ....

Temperature: .... Pulse: ....

Respiration: .... Blood pressure: ....

2. Obstetrical Examination:

a. Breast Examination:

Size and shape: .... Sensation: ....

Primary areola: .... Secondary areola: ....

Montgomery tubercles: .... Colostrums: ....

Nipples: ....

b. Abdominal Examination:

Inspection: ....

Size of the abdomen: .... Shape of the abdomen: ....

Contour of the abdominal wall:

- Skin changes on the abdomen: ....
- Previous operation scar: ....
- Striae gravidarum: ....
- Linea nigra: ....
- Umbilicus: Flattened/Protruded/Dimpled.

Visible fetal movement: ....

Flank region/Filled/Empty

Appearance of the skin infection: ....

Fundal Height (in cm): .... Abdominal girth (in cm): ....

- Abdominal palpation:

Fundal palpation: ....

Lateral palpation: ....

(i) Right lateral palpation: ....

(ii) Left lateral palpation: ....

Pelvic Palpation: ....

Pawlik's grip: ....

Auscultation: ....

- Findings:

Lie: .... Attitude: ....

Presentation: .... Position: ....

Denominator: ....

- Vaginal examination:

Discharge: .... Normal: ....

Abnormal: .... Foul smelling: ....

(VDRL) infection: ....

Investigation done

Date	*Investigation Done*	*Mothers Value*	*Normal Value*	*Remarks*

Any other specific investigation: ....

- Treatment Given: ....

....

....

....

....

Name of the Drug	*Dosag/Route/Frequency*	*Action*	*Side Effects*	*Nurses Responsibility*

Sl No.	*Needs Identified*	*Nursing Care Given*

- Antenatal advices: ....
  ....
  ....
  ....
  ....

General health condition of the mother: ....

Signature of the Student

Signature of the Supervisor

NURSING CARE PLAN

Assessment	*Nursing Diagnosis*	*Goals*	*Nursing Intervention*	*Rationale*	*Nursing Implementation*	*Evaluation*

NURSING CARE PLAN

Assessment	*Nursing Diagnosis*	*Goals*	*Nursing Intervention*	*Rationale*	*Nursing Implementation*	*Evaluation*

NURSING CARE PLAN

Assessment	*Nursing Diagnosis*	*Goals*	*Nursing Intervention*	*Rationale*	*Nursing Implementation*	*Evaluation*

ANTENATAL EXAMINATION (3)

HISTORY COLLECTION

1. Baseline Data:

Name of the Mother: .... Date of Registration: ....

Age: .... Date of Admission: ....

Religion: .... Date of Assessment: ....

Hospital Number: .... Procedure Performed: ....

[Wards, Primary health center (PHC), Out patient department (OPD), Home]

Marital Status: ....

LMP: ....

EDD: ....

Period of gestation: ....

Obstetrical score:

G		P		L		A		S		D	

G-Gravida: .... P-Para: ....

L-Living: .... A-Abortion: ....

S-Still birth: .... D-Death: ....

Diagnosis: ....

Address: ....

2. Socioeconomic History:

Educational Status: .... Husband: ....

Wife: ....

Occupation: .... Husband: ....

Wife: ....

Total income: ....

Type of house: ....

Living standard:

Ownership of the house: Own house/Rented house

Lighting facility: ....

Environmental conditions of the house: Water facility: ....

Toilet facility: ....

Drainage, kitchen, garden: ....

Pet animals: ....

Cultural background: ....

3. Family History:

Sl No.	Name of the Family Member	Age	Sex	Educational Status	Occupation	Relationship with the Mother	Health Status
1.							
2.							
3.							
4.							
5.							
6.							

History of any

- Communicable diseases: ....
- Hereditary diseases: ....
- Twin pregnancy: ....
- Bad obstetrical history: ....

4. Personal History:
   - Dietary pattern: ....
   - Sleeping pattern: ....
   - Habits: ....
   - Bowel elimination: ....
   - Bladder elimination: ....
   - Immunization history: ....
   - Sexual history: ....
   - Drug history/Drug allergy: ....

5. Menstrual History: ....

....

6. Marital History: ....

....

7. Contraceptive History: ....

....

8. Previous Medical and Surgical History: ....

....

9. Previous Obstetrical History:

Sl No.	*Year*	*Antenatal Period*	*Intranatal Period*	*Postnatal Period*	*Alive/ Stillbirth*	*Sex*	*Weight*	*Remarks*
1								
2								
3								
4								
5								
6								

10. Present Obstetrical History:

a. Antenatal: ....

....

....

b. Intranatal: ....

....

....

c. Postnatal: ....

....

....

ANTENATAL EXAMINATION

1. General Examination:

General appearance: .... Psychological status: ....

Head: .... Hair: ....

Facial appearance: .... Eyes: ....

Ears: .... Nose: ....

Mouth: .... Mucus membranes: ....

Gums: .... Teeth: ....

Tongue: .... Tonsils: ....

Neck: .... Upper limbs: ....

Chest: .... Lungs: ....

Heart: .... Lower limbs: ....

Back: .... Vital signs: ....

Temperature: .... Pulse: ....

Respiration: .... Blood pressure: ....

2. Obstetrical Examination:

   a. Breast Examination:

   Size and shape: .... Sensation: ....

   Primary areola: .... Secondary areola: ....

   Montgomery tubercles: .... Colostrums: ....

   Nipples: ....

   b. Abdominal Examination:

   Inspection: ....

   Size of the abdomen: .... Shape of the abdomen: ....

   Contour of the abdominal wall:

   - Skin changes on the abdomen: ....
   - Previous operation scar: ....
   - Striae gravidarum: ....
   - Linea nigra: ....
   - Umbilicus: Flattened/Protruded/Dimpled.

     Visible fetal movement: ....

     Flank region/Filled/Empty

Appearance of the skin infection: ....

Fundal Height (in cm): .... Abdominal girth (in cm): ....

- Abdominal palpation:

Fundal palpation: ....

Lateral palpation: ....

(i) Right lateral palpation: ....

(ii) Left lateral palpation: ....

Pelvic Palpation: ....

Pawlik's grip: ....

Auscultation: ....

- Findings:

Lie: .... Attitude: ....

Presentation: .... Position: ....

Denominator: ....

- Vaginal examination:

Discharge: .... Normal: ....

Abnormal: .... Foul smelling: ....

(VDRL) infection: ....

Investigation done

Date	*Investigation Done*	*Mothers Value*	*Normal Value*	*Remarks*

Any other specific investigation: ....

- Treatment Given: ....

....

....

....

....

Name of the Drug	*Dosag/Route/Frequency*	*Action*	*Side Effects*	*Nurses Responsibility*

Sl No.	*Needs Identified*	*Nursing Care Given*

- Antenatal advices: ....

....

....

....

....

General health condition of the mother: ....

Signature of the Student

Signature of the Supervisor

NURSING CARE PLAN

Assessment	*Nursing Diagnosis*	*Goals*	*Nursing Intervention*	*Rationale*	*Nursing Implementation*	*Evaluation*

NURSING CARE PLAN

Assessment	*Nursing Diagnosis*	*Goals*	*Nursing Intervention*	*Rationale*	*Nursing Implementation*	*Evaluation*

NURSING CARE PLAN

Assessment	*Nursing Diagnosis*	*Goals*	*Nursing Intervention*	*Rationale*	*Nursing Implementation*	*Evaluation*

ANTENATAL EXAMINATION (4)

HISTORY COLLECTION

1. Baseline Data:

Name of the Mother: ....

Date of Registration: ....

Age: ....

Date of Admission: ....

Religion: ....

Date of Assessment: ....

Hospital Number: ....

Procedure Performed: ....

[Wards, Primary health center (PHC), Out patient department (OPD), Home]

Marital Status: ....

LMP: ....

EDD: ....

Period of gestation: ....

Obstetrical score:

G		P		L		A		S		D	

G-Gravida: ....

P-Para: ....

L-Living: ....

A-Abortion: ....

S-Still birth: ....

D-Death: ....

Diagnosis: ....

Address: ....

2. Socioeconomic History:

Educational Status: ....

Husband: ....

Wife: ....

Occupation: ....

Husband: ....

Wife: ....

Total income: ....

Type of house: ....

Living standard:

Ownership of the house: Own house/Rented house

Lighting facility: ....

Environmental conditions of the house:

Water facility: ....

Toilet facility: ....

Drainage, kitchen, garden: ....

Pet animals: ....

Cultural background: ....

3. Family History:

Sl No.	*Name of the Family Member*	*Age*	*Sex*	*Educational Status*	*Occupation*	*Relationship with the Mother*	*Health Status*
1.							
2.							
3.							
4.							
5.							
6.							

History of any

- Communicable diseases: ....
- Hereditary diseases: ....
- Twin pregnancy: ....
- Bad obstetrical history: ....

4. Personal History:
   - Dietary pattern: ....
   - Sleeping pattern: ....
   - Habits: ....
   - Bowel elimination: ....
   - Bladder elimination: ....
   - Immunization history: ....
   - Sexual history: ....
   - Drug history/Drug allergy: ....

5. Menstrual History: ....

....

6. Marital History: ....

....

7. Contraceptive History: ....

....

8. Previous Medical and Surgical History: ....

....

9. Previous Obstetrical History:

Sl No.	*Year*	*Antenatal Period*	*Intranatal Period*	*Postnatal Period*	*Alive/ Stillbirth*	*Sex*	*Weight*	*Remarks*
1								
2								
3								
4								
5								
6								

10. Present Obstetrical History:

    a. Antenatal: ....

    ....

    ....

    b. Intranatal: ....

    ....

    ....

    c. Postnatal: ....

    ....

    ....

ANTENATAL EXAMINATION

1. General Examination:

General appearance: .... Psychological status: ....

Head: .... Hair: ....

Facial appearance: .... Eyes: ....

Ears: .... Nose: ....

Mouth: .... Mucus membranes: ....

Gums: .... Teeth: ....

Tongue: .... Tonsils: ....

Neck: .... Upper limbs: ....

Chest: .... Lungs: ....

Heart: .... Lower limbs: ....

Back: .... Vital signs: ....

Temperature: .... Pulse: ....

Respiration: .... Blood pressure: ....

2. Obstetrical Examination:

a. Breast Examination:

Size and shape: .... Sensation: ....

Primary areola: .... Secondary areola: ....

Montgomery tubercles: .... Colostrums: ....

Nipples: ....

b. Abdominal Examination:

Inspection: ....

Size of the abdomen: .... Shape of the abdomen: ....

Contour of the abdominal wall:

- Skin changes on the abdomen: ....
- Previous operation scar: ....
- Striae gravidarum: ....
- Linea nigra: ....
- Umbilicus: Flattened/Protruded/Dimpled.

Visible fetal movement: ....

Flank region/Filled/Empty

Appearance of the skin infection: ....

Fundal Height (in cm): .... Abdominal girth (in cm): ....

- Abdominal palpation:

Fundal palpation: ....

Lateral palpation: ....

(i) Right lateral palpation: ....

(ii) Left lateral palpation: ....

Pelvic Palpation: ....

Pawlik's grip: ....

Auscultation: ....

- Findings:

Lie: .... Attitude: ....

Presentation: .... Position: ....

Denominator: ....

- Vaginal examination:

Discharge: .... Normal: ....

Abnormal: .... Foul smelling: ....

(VDRL) infection: ....

Investigation done

Date	*Investigation Done*	*Mothers Value*	*Normal Value*	*Remarks*

Any other specific investigation: ....

- Treatment Given: ....

....

....

....

....

Name of the Drug	*Dosag/Route/Frequency*	*Action*	*Side Effects*	*Nurses Responsibility*

Sl No.	*Needs Identified*	*Nursing Care Given*

- Antenatal advices: ....

....

....

....

....

General health condition of the mother: ....

Signature of the Student

Signature of the Supervisor

NURSING CARE PLAN

Assessment	*Nursing Diagnosis*	*Goals*	*Nursing Intervention*	*Rationale*	*Nursing Implementation*	*Evaluation*

NURSING CARE PLAN

Assessment	*Nursing Diagnosis*	*Goals*	*Nursing Intervention*	*Rationale*	*Nursing Implementation*	*Evaluation*

NURSING CARE PLAN

Assessment	*Nursing Diagnosis*	*Goals*	*Nursing Intervention*	*Rationale*	*Nursing Implementation*	*Evaluation*

ANTENATAL EXAMINATION (5)

HISTORY COLLECTION

1. Baseline Data:

Name of the Mother: .... Date of Registration: ....

Age: .... Date of Admission: ....

Religion: .... Date of Assessment: ....

Hospital Number: .... Procedure Performed: ....

[Wards, Primary health center (PHC), Out patient department (OPD), Home]

Marital Status: ....

LMP: ....

EDD: ....

Period of gestation: ....

Obstetrical score:

G		P		L		A		S		D	

G-Gravida: .... P-Para: ....

L-Living: .... A-Abortion: ....

S-Still birth: .... D-Death: ....

Diagnosis: ....

Address: ....

2. Socioeconomic History:

Educational Status: .... Husband: ....

Wife: ....

Occupation: .... Husband: ....

Wife: ....

Total income: ....

Type of house: ....

Living standard:

Ownership of the house: Own house/Rented house

Lighting facility: ....

Environmental conditions of the house: Water facility: ....

Toilet facility: ....

Drainage, kitchen, garden: ....

Pet animals: ....

Cultural background: ....

3. Family History:

Sl No.	*Name of the Family Member*	*Age*	*Sex*	*Educational Status*	*Occupation*	*Relationship with the Mother*	*Health Status*
1.							
2.							
3.							
4.							
5.							
6.							

History of any

- Communicable diseases: ....
- Hereditary diseases: ....
- Twin pregnancy: ....
- Bad obstetrical history: ....

4. Personal History:
   - Dietary pattern: ....
   - Sleeping pattern: ....
   - Habits: ....
   - Bowel elimination: ....
   - Bladder elimination: ....
   - Immunization history: ....
   - Sexual history: ....
   - Drug history/Drug allergy: ....

5. Menstrual History: ....

....

6. Marital History: ....

....

7. Contraceptive History: ....

....

8. Previous Medical and Surgical History: ....

....

9. Previous Obstetrical History:

Sl No.	*Year*	*Antenatal Period*	*Intranatal Period*	*Postnatal Period*	*Alive/ Stillbirth*	*Sex*	*Weight*	*Remarks*
1								
2								
3								
4								
5								
6								

10. Present Obstetrical History:

    a. Antenatal: ....

    ....

    ....

    b. Intranatal: ....

    ....

    ....

    c. Postnatal: ....

    ....

    ....

ANTENATAL EXAMINATION

1. General Examination:

General appearance: .... Psychological status: ....

Head: .... Hair: ....

Facial appearance: .... Eyes: ....

Ears: .... Nose: ....

Mouth: .... Mucus membranes: ....

Gums: .... Teeth: ....

Tongue: .... Tonsils: ....

Neck: .... Upper limbs: ....

Chest: .... Lungs: ....

Heart: .... Lower limbs: ....

Back: .... Vital signs: ....

Temperature: .... Pulse: ....

Respiration: .... Blood pressure: ....

2. Obstetrical Examination:

a. Breast Examination:

Size and shape: .... Sensation: ....

Primary areola: .... Secondary areola: ....

Montgomery tubercles: .... Colostrums: ....

Nipples: ....

b. Abdominal Examination:

Inspection: ....

Size of the abdomen: .... Shape of the abdomen: ....

Contour of the abdominal wall:

- Skin changes on the abdomen: ....
- Previous operation scar: ....
- Striae gravidarum: ....
- Linea nigra: ....
- Umbilicus: Flattened/Protruded/Dimpled.

Visible fetal movement: ....

Flank region/Filled/Empty

Appearance of the skin infection: ....

Fundal Height (in cm): .... Abdominal girth (in cm): ....

- Abdominal palpation:

Fundal palpation: ....

Lateral palpation: ....

(i) Right lateral palpation: ....

(ii) Left lateral palpation: ....

Pelvic Palpation: ....

Pawlik's grip: ....

Auscultation: ....

- Findings:

Lie: .... Attitude: ....

Presentation: .... Position: ....

Denominator: ....

- Vaginal examination:

Discharge: .... Normal: ....

Abnormal: .... Foul smelling: ....

(VDRL) infection: ....

Investigation done

Date	*Investigation Done*	*Mothers Value*	*Normal Value*	*Remarks*

Any other specific investigation: ....

- Treatment Given: ....

....

....

....

....

Name of the Drug	*Dosag/Route/Frequency*	*Action*	*Side Effects*	*Nurses Responsibility*

Sl No.	*Needs Identified*	*Nursing Care Given*

- Antenatal advices: ....
....
....
....
....

General health condition of the mother: ....

Signature of the Student

Signature of the Supervisor

NURSING CARE PLAN

Assessment	*Nursing Diagnosis*	*Goals*	*Nursing Intervention*	*Rationale*	*Nursing Implementation*	*Evaluation*

NURSING CARE PLAN

Assessment	*Nursing Diagnosis*	*Goals*	*Nursing Intervention*	*Rationale*	*Nursing Implementation*	*Evaluation*

NURSING CARE PLAN

Assessment	Nursing Diagnosis	Goals	Nursing Intervention	Rationale	Nursing Implementation	Evaluation

ANTENATAL EXAMINATION (6)

HISTORY COLLECTION

1. Baseline Data:

Name of the Mother: .... Date of Registration: ....

Age: .... Date of Admission: ....

Religion: .... Date of Assessment: ....

Hospital Number: .... Procedure Performed: ....

[Wards, Primary health center (PHC), Out patient department (OPD), Home]

Marital Status: ....

LMP: ....

EDD: ....

Period of gestation: ....

Obstetrical score:

G		P		L		A		S		D	

G-Gravida: .... P-Para: ....

L-Living: .... A-Abortion: ....

S-Still birth: .... D-Death: ....

Diagnosis: ....

Address: ....

2. Socioeconomic History:

Educational Status: .... Husband: ....

Wife: ....

Occupation: .... Husband: ....

Wife: ....

Total income: ....

Type of house: ....

Living standard:

Ownership of the house: Own house/Rented house

Lighting facility: ....

Environmental conditions of the house: Water facility: ....

Toilet facility: ....

Drainage, kitchen, garden: ....

Pet animals: ....

Cultural background: ....

3. Family History:

Sl No.	*Name of the Family Member*	*Age*	*Sex*	*Educational Status*	*Occupation*	*Relationship with the Mother*	*Health Status*
1.							
2.							
3.							
4.							
5.							
6.							

History of any

- Communicable diseases: ....
- Hereditary diseases: ....
- Twin pregnancy: ....
- Bad obstetrical history: ....

4. Personal History:
   - Dietary pattern: ....
   - Sleeping pattern: ....
   - Habits: ....
   - Bowel elimination: ....
   - Bladder elimination: ....
   - Immunization history: ....
   - Sexual history: ....
   - Drug history/Drug allergy: ....

5. Menstrual History: ....

....

6. Marital History: ....

....

7. Contraceptive History: ....

....

8. Previous Medical and Surgical History: ....

....

9. Previous Obstetrical History:

Sl No.	*Year*	*Antenatal Period*	*Intranatal Period*	*Postnatal Period*	*Alive/ Stillbirth*	*Sex*	*Weight*	*Remarks*
1								
2								
3								
4								
5								
6								

10. Present Obstetrical History:

    a. Antenatal: ....

    ....

    ....

    b. Intranatal: ....

    ....

    ....

    c. Postnatal: ....

    ....

    ....

ANTENATAL EXAMINATION

1. General Examination:

   General appearance: ....

   Psychological status: ....

   Head: ....

   Hair: ....

   Facial appearance: ....

   Eyes: ....

   Ears: ....

   Nose: ....

   Mouth: ....

   Mucus membranes: ....

   Gums: ....

   Teeth: ....

   Tongue: ....

   Tonsils: ....

   Neck: ....

   Upper limbs: ....

   Chest: ....

   Lungs: ....

   Heart: ....

   Lower limbs: ....

   Back: ....

   Vital signs: ....

   Temperature: ....

   Pulse: ....

   Respiration: ....

   Blood pressure: ....

2. Obstetrical Examination:

   a. Breast Examination:

      Size and shape: ....

      Sensation: ....

      Primary areola: ....

      Secondary areola: ....

      Montgomery tubercles: ....

      Colostrums: ....

      Nipples: ....

   b. Abdominal Examination:

      Inspection: ....

      Size of the abdomen: ....

      Shape of the abdomen: ....

      Contour of the abdominal wall:

      - Skin changes on the abdomen: ....
      - Previous operation scar: ....
      - Striae gravidarum: ....
      - Linea nigra: ....
      - Umbilicus: Flattened/Protruded/Dimpled.

        Visible fetal movement: ....

        Flank region/Filled/Empty

Appearance of the skin infection: ....

Fundal Height (in cm): .... Abdominal girth (in cm): ....

- Abdominal palpation:

Fundal palpation: ....

Lateral palpation: ....

(i) Right lateral palpation: ....

(ii) Left lateral palpation: ....

Pelvic Palpation: ....

Pawlik's grip: ....

Auscultation: ....

- Findings:

Lie: .... Attitude: ....

Presentation: .... Position: ....

Denominator: ....

- Vaginal examination:

Discharge: .... Normal: ....

Abnormal: .... Foul smelling: ....

(VDRL) infection: ....

Investigation done

Date	*Investigation Done*	*Mothers Value*	*Normal Value*	*Remarks*

Any other specific investigation: ....

- Treatment Given: ....

....

....

....

....

Name of the Drug	*Dosag/Route/Frequency*	*Action*	*Side Effects*	*Nurses Responsibility*

Sl No.	*Needs Identified*	*Nursing Care Given*

- Antenatal advices: ....
....
....
....
....

General health condition of the mother: ....

Signature of the Student

Signature of the Supervisor

NURSING CARE PLAN

Assessment	*Nursing Diagnosis*	*Goals*	*Nursing Intervention*	*Rationale*	*Nursing Implementation*	*Evaluation*

NURSING CARE PLAN

Assessment	*Nursing Diagnosis*	*Goals*	*Nursing Intervention*	*Rationale*	*Nursing Implementation*	*Evaluation*

NURSING CARE PLAN

Assessment	*Nursing Diagnosis*	*Goals*	*Nursing Intervention*	*Rationale*	*Nursing Implementation*	*Evaluation*

ANTENATAL EXAMINATION (7)

HISTORY COLLECTION

1. Baseline Data:

Name of the Mother: .... Date of Registration: ....

Age: .... Date of Admission: ....

Religion: .... Date of Assessment: ....

Hospital Number: .... Procedure Performed: ....

[Wards, Primary health center (PHC), Out patient department (OPD), Home]

Marital Status: ....

LMP: ....

EDD: ....

Period of gestation: ....

Obstetrical score:

G		P		L		A		S		D	

G-Gravida: .... P-Para: ....

L-Living: .... A-Abortion: ....

S-Still birth: .... D-Death: ....

Diagnosis: ....

Address: ....

2. Socioeconomic History:

Educational Status: .... Husband: ....

Wife: ....

Occupation: .... Husband: ....

Wife: ....

Total income: ....

Type of house: ....

Living standard:

Ownership of the house: Own house/Rented house

Lighting facility: ....

Environmental conditions of the house: Water facility: ....

Toilet facility: ....

Drainage, kitchen, garden: ....

Pet animals: ....

Cultural background: ....

3. Family History:

Sl No.	*Name of the Family Member*	*Age*	*Sex*	*Educational Status*	*Occupation*	*Relationship with the Mother*	*Health Status*
1.							
2.							
3.							
4.							
5.							
6.							

History of any

- Communicable diseases: ....
- Hereditary diseases: ....
- Twin pregnancy: ....
- Bad obstetrical history: ....

4. Personal History:
   - Dietary pattern: ....
   - Sleeping pattern: ....
   - Habits: ....
   - Bowel elimination: ....
   - Bladder elimination: ....
   - Immunization history: ....
   - Sexual history: ....
   - Drug history/Drug allergy: ....

5. Menstrual History: ....

....

6. Marital History: ....

....

7. Contraceptive History: ....

....

8. Previous Medical and Surgical History: ....

....

9. Previous Obstetrical History:

Sl No.	*Year*	*Antenatal Period*	*Intranatal Period*	*Postnatal Period*	*Alive/ Stillbirth*	*Sex*	*Weight*	*Remarks*
1								
2								
3								
4								
5								
6								

10. Present Obstetrical History:

a. Antenatal: ....

....

....

b. Intranatal: ....

....

....

c. Postnatal: ....

....

....

ANTENATAL EXAMINATION

1. General Examination:

General appearance: ....

Psychological status: ....

Head: ....

Hair: ....

Facial appearance: ....

Eyes: ....

Ears: ....

Nose: ....

Mouth: ....

Mucus membranes: ....

Gums: ....

Teeth: ....

Tongue: ....

Tonsils: ....

Neck: ....

Upper limbs: ....

Chest: ....

Lungs: ....

Heart: ....

Lower limbs: ....

Back: ....

Vital signs: ....

Temperature: ....

Pulse: ....

Respiration: ....

Blood pressure: ....

2. Obstetrical Examination:

a. Breast Examination:

Size and shape: ....

Sensation: ....

Primary areola: ....

Secondary areola: ....

Montgomery tubercles: ....

Colostrums: ....

Nipples: ....

b. Abdominal Examination:

Inspection: ....

Size of the abdomen: ....

Shape of the abdomen: ....

Contour of the abdominal wall:

- Skin changes on the abdomen: ....
- Previous operation scar: ....
- Striae gravidarum: ....
- Linea nigra: ....
- Umbilicus: Flattened/Protruded/Dimpled.

Visible fetal movement: ....

Flank region/Filled/Empty

Appearance of the skin infection: ....

Fundal Height (in cm): .... Abdominal girth (in cm): ....

- Abdominal palpation:

Fundal palpation: ....

Lateral palpation: ....

(i) Right lateral palpation: ....

(ii) Left lateral palpation: ....

Pelvic Palpation: ....

Pawlik's grip: ....

- Auscultation: ....
- Findings:

Lie: .... Attitude: ....

Presentation: .... Position: ....

Denominator: ....

- Vaginal examination:

Discharge: .... Normal: ....

Abnormal: .... Foul smelling: ....

(VDRL) infection: ....

Investigation done

Date	*Investigation Done*	*Mothers Value*	*Normal Value*	*Remarks*

Any other specific investigation: ....

- Treatment Given: ....

....

....

....

....

Name of the Drug	*Dosag/Route/Frequency*	*Action*	*Side Effects*	*Nurses Responsibility*

Sl No.	*Needs Identified*	*Nursing Care Given*

- Antenatal advices: ....

....

....

....

....

General health condition of the mother: ....

Signature of the Student

Signature of the Supervisor

NURSING CARE PLAN

Assessment	*Nursing Diagnosis*	*Goals*	*Nursing Intervention*	*Rationale*	*Nursing Implementation*	*Evaluation*

NURSING CARE PLAN

Assessment	*Nursing Diagnosis*	*Goals*	*Nursing Intervention*	*Rationale*	*Nursing Implementation*	*Evaluation*

NURSING CARE PLAN

Assessment	*Nursing Diagnosis*	*Goals*	*Nursing Intervention*	*Rationale*	*Nursing Implementation*	*Evaluation*

ANTENATAL EXAMINATION (8)

HISTORY COLLECTION

1. Baseline Data:

Name of the Mother: .... Date of Registration: ....

Age: .... Date of Admission: ....

Religion: .... Date of Assessment: ....

Hospital Number: .... Procedure Performed: ....

[Wards, Primary health center (PHC), Out patient department (OPD), Home]

Marital Status: ....

LMP: ....

EDD: ....

Period of gestation: ....

Obstetrical score:

G		P		L		A		S		D	

G-Gravida: .... P-Para: ....

L-Living: .... A-Abortion: ....

S-Still birth: .... D-Death: ....

Diagnosis: ....

Address: ....

2. Socioeconomic History:

Educational Status: .... Husband: ....

Wife: ....

Occupation: .... Husband: ....

Wife: ....

Total income: ....

Type of house: ....

Living standard:

Ownership of the house: Own house/Rented house

Lighting facility: ....

Environmental conditions of the house: Water facility: ....

Toilet facility: ....

Drainage, kitchen, garden: ....

Pet animals: ....

Cultural background: ....

3. Family History:

Sl No.	*Name of the Family Member*	*Age*	*Sex*	*Educational Status*	*Occupation*	*Relationship with the Mother*	*Health Status*
1.							
2.							
3.							
4.							
5.							
6.							

History of any

- Communicable diseases: ....
- Hereditary diseases: ....
- Twin pregnancy: ....
- Bad obstetrical history: ....

4. Personal History:

- Dietary pattern: ....
- Sleeping pattern: ....
- Habits: ....
- Bowel elimination: ....
- Bladder elimination: ....
- Immunization history: ....
- Sexual history: ....
- Drug history/Drug allergy: ....

5. Menstrual History: ....

....

6. Marital History: ....

....

7. Contraceptive History: ....

....

8. Previous Medical and Surgical History: ....

....

9. Previous Obstetrical History:

Sl No.	*Year*	*Antenatal Period*	*Intranatal Period*	*Postnatal Period*	*Alive/ Stillbirth*	*Sex*	*Weight*	*Remarks*
1								
2								
3								
4								
5								
6								

10. Present Obstetrical History:

    a. Antenatal: ....

    ....

    ....

    b. Intranatal: ....

    ....

    ....

    c. Postnatal: ....

    ....

    ....

ANTENATAL EXAMINATION

1. General Examination:

General appearance: ....

Psychological status: ....

Head: ....

Hair: ....

Facial appearance: ....

Eyes: ....

Ears: ....

Nose: ....

Mouth: ....

Mucus membranes: ....

Gums: ....

Teeth: ....

Tongue: ....

Tonsils: ....

Neck: ....

Upper limbs: ....

Chest: ....

Lungs: ....

Heart: ....

Lower limbs: ....

Back: ....

Vital signs: ....

Temperature: ....

Pulse: ....

Respiration: ....

Blood pressure: ....

2. Obstetrical Examination:

a. Breast Examination:

Size and shape: ....

Sensation: ....

Primary areola: ....

Secondary areola: ....

Montgomery tubercles: ....

Colostrums: ....

Nipples: ....

b. Abdominal Examination:

Inspection: ....

Size of the abdomen: ....

Shape of the abdomen: ....

Contour of the abdominal wall:

- Skin changes on the abdomen: ....
- Previous operation scar: ....
- Striae gravidarum: ....
- Linea nigra: ....
- Umbilicus: Flattened/Protruded/Dimpled.

Visible fetal movement: ....

Flank region/Filled/Empty

Appearance of the skin infection: ....

Fundal Height (in cm): .... Abdominal girth (in cm): ....

- Abdominal palpation:

Fundal palpation: ....

Lateral palpation: ....

(i) Right lateral palpation: ....

(ii) Left lateral palpation: ....

Pelvic Palpation: ....

Pawlik's grip: ....

Auscultation: ....

- Findings:

Lie: .... Attitude: ....

Presentation: .... Position: ....

Denominator: ....

- Vaginal examination:

Discharge: .... Normal: ....

Abnormal: .... Foul smelling: ....

(VDRL) infection: ....

Investigation done

Date	*Investigation Done*	*Mothers Value*	*Normal Value*	*Remarks*

Any other specific investigation: ....

- Treatment Given: ....

....

....

....

....

Name of the Drug	*Dosag/Route/Frequency*	*Action*	*Side Effects*	*Nurses Responsibility*

Sl No.	*Needs Identified*	*Nursing Care Given*

- Antenatal advices: ....
....
....
....
....

General health condition of the mother: ....

Signature of the Student

Signature of the Supervisor

NURSING CARE PLAN

Assessment	*Nursing Diagnosis*	*Goals*	*Nursing Intervention*	*Rationale*	*Nursing Implementation*	*Evaluation*

NURSING CARE PLAN

Assessment	*Nursing Diagnosis*	*Goals*	*Nursing Intervention*	*Rationale*	*Nursing Implementation*	*Evaluation*

NURSING CARE PLAN

Assessment	*Nursing Diagnosis*	*Goals*	*Nursing Intervention*	*Rationale*	*Nursing Implementation*	*Evaluation*

ANTENATAL EXAMINATION (9)

HISTORY COLLECTION

1. Baseline Data:

Name of the Mother: ....

Date of Registration: ....

Age: ....

Date of Admission: ....

Religion: ....

Date of Assessment: ....

Hospital Number: ....

Procedure Performed: ....

[Wards, Primary health center (PHC), Out patient department (OPD), Home]

Marital Status: ....

LMP: ....

EDD: ....

Period of gestation: ....

Obstetrical score:

G		P		L		A		S		D	

G-Gravida: ....

P-Para: ....

L-Living: ....

A-Abortion: ....

S-Still birth: ....

D-Death: ....

Diagnosis: ....

Address: ....

2. Socioeconomic History:

Educational Status: ....

Husband: ....

Wife: ....

Occupation: ....

Husband: ....

Wife: ....

Total income: ....

Type of house: ....

Living standard:

Ownership of the house: Own house/Rented house

Lighting facility: ....

Environmental conditions of the house:

Water facility: ....

Toilet facility: ....

Drainage, kitchen, garden: ....

Pet animals: ....

Cultural background: ....

3. Family History:

Sl No.	*Name of the Family Member*	*Age*	*Sex*	*Educational Status*	*Occupation*	*Relationship with the Mother*	*Health Status*
1.							
2.							
3.							
4.							
5.							
6.							

History of any

- Communicable diseases: ....
- Hereditary diseases: ....
- Twin pregnancy: ....
- Bad obstetrical history: ....

4. Personal History:
   - Dietary pattern: ....
   - Sleeping pattern: ....
   - Habits: ....
   - Bowel elimination: ....
   - Bladder elimination: ....
   - Immunization history: ....
   - Sexual history: ....
   - Drug history/Drug allergy: ....
5. Menstrual History: ....

....

6. Marital History: ....

....

7. Contraceptive History: ....

....

8. Previous Medical and Surgical History: ....

....

9. Previous Obstetrical History:

Sl No.	*Year*	*Antenatal Period*	*Intranatal Period*	*Postnatal Period*	*Alive/ Stillbirth*	*Sex*	*Weight*	*Remarks*
1								
2								
3								
4								
5								
6								

10. Present Obstetrical History:

    a. Antenatal: ....

    ....

    ....

    b. Intranatal: ....

    ....

    ....

    c. Postnatal: ....

    ....

    ....

ANTENATAL EXAMINATION

1. General Examination:

General appearance: ....

Psychological status: ....

Head: ....

Hair: ....

Facial appearance: ....

Eyes: ....

Ears: ....

Nose: ....

Mouth: ....

Mucus membranes: ....

Gums: ....

Teeth: ....

Tongue: ....

Tonsils: ....

Neck: ....

Upper limbs: ....

Chest: ....

Lungs: ....

Heart: ....

Lower limbs: ....

Back: ....

Vital signs: ....

Temperature: ....

Pulse: ....

Respiration: ....

Blood pressure: ....

2. Obstetrical Examination:

a. Breast Examination:

Size and shape: ....

Sensation: ....

Primary areola: ....

Secondary areola: ....

Montgomery tubercles: ....

Colostrums: ....

Nipples: ....

b. Abdominal Examination:

Inspection: ....

Size of the abdomen: ....

Shape of the abdomen: ....

Contour of the abdominal wall:

- Skin changes on the abdomen: ....
- Previous operation scar: ....
- Striae gravidarum: ....
- Linea nigra: ....
- Umbilicus: Flattened/Protruded/Dimpled.

Visible fetal movement: ....

Flank region/Filled/Empty

Appearance of the skin infection: ....

Fundal Height (in cm): .... Abdominal girth (in cm): ....

- Abdominal palpation:

Fundal palpation: ....

Lateral palpation: ....

(i) Right lateral palpation: ....

(ii) Left lateral palpation: ....

Pelvic Palpation: ....

Pawlik's grip: ....

Auscultation: ....

- Findings:

Lie: .... Attitude: ....

Presentation: .... Position: ....

Denominator: ....

- Vaginal examination:

Discharge: .... Normal: ....

Abnormal: .... Foul smelling: ....

(VDRL) infection: ....

Investigation done

Date	*Investigation Done*	*Mothers Value*	*Normal Value*	*Remarks*

Any other specific investigation: ....

- Treatment Given: ....

....

....

....

....

Name of the Drug	*Dosag/Route/Frequency*	*Action*	*Side Effects*	*Nurses Responsibility*

Sl No.	*Needs Identified*	*Nursing Care Given*

- Antenatal advices: ....

....

....

....

....

General health condition of the mother: ....

Signature of the Student

Signature of the Supervisor

NURSING CARE PLAN

Assessment	*Nursing Diagnosis*	*Goals*	*Nursing Intervention*	*Rationale*	*Nursing Implementation*	*Evaluation*

NURSING CARE PLAN

Assessment	*Nursing Diagnosis*	*Goals*	*Nursing Intervention*	*Rationale*	*Nursing Implementation*	*Evaluation*

NURSING CARE PLAN

Assessment	*Nursing Diagnosis*	*Goals*	*Nursing Intervention*	*Rationale*	*Nursing Implementation*	*Evaluation*

ANTENATAL EXAMINATION (10)

HISTORY COLLECTION

1. Baseline Data:

Name of the Mother: .... Date of Registration: ....

Age: .... Date of Admission: ....

Religion: .... Date of Assessment: ....

Hospital Number: .... Procedure Performed: ....

[Wards, Primary health center (PHC), Out patient department (OPD), Home]

Marital Status: ....

LMP: ....

EDD: ....

Period of gestation: ....

Obstetrical score:

G		P		L		A		S		D	

G-Gravida: .... P-Para: ....

L-Living: .... A-Abortion: ....

S-Still birth: .... D-Death: ....

Diagnosis: ....

Address: ....

2. Socioeconomic History:

Educational Status: .... Husband: ....

Wife: ....

Occupation: .... Husband: ....

Wife: ....

Total income: ....

Type of house: ....

Living standard:

Ownership of the house: Own house/Rented house

Lighting facility: ....

Environmental conditions of the house: Water facility: ....

Toilet facility: ....

Drainage, kitchen, garden: ....

Pet animals: ....

Cultural background: ....

3. Family History:

Sl No.	*Name of the Family Member*	*Age*	*Sex*	*Educational Status*	*Occupation*	*Relationship with the Mother*	*Health Status*
1.							
2.							
3.							
4.							
5.							
6.							

History of any

- Communicable diseases: ....
- Hereditary diseases: ....
- Twin pregnancy: ....
- Bad obstetrical history: ....

4. Personal History:
   - Dietary pattern: ....
   - Sleeping pattern: ....
   - Habits: ....
   - Bowel elimination: ....
   - Bladder elimination: ....
   - Immunization history: ....
   - Sexual history: ....
   - Drug history/Drug allergy: ....

5. Menstrual History: ....

....

6. Marital History: ....

....

7. Contraceptive History: ....

....

8. Previous Medical and Surgical History: ....

....

9. Previous Obstetrical History:

Sl No.	*Year*	*Antenatal Period*	*Intranatal Period*	*Postnatal Period*	*Alive/ Stillbirth*	*Sex*	*Weight*	*Remarks*
1								
2								
3								
4								
5								
6								

10. Present Obstetrical History:

    a. Antenatal: ....

    ....

    ....

    b. Intranatal: ....

    ....

    ....

    c. Postnatal: ....

    ....

    ....

ANTENATAL EXAMINATION

1. General Examination:

General appearance: ....

Psychological status: ....

Head: ....

Hair: ....

Facial appearance: ....

Eyes: ....

Ears: ....

Nose: ....

Mouth: ....

Mucus membranes: ....

Gums: ....

Teeth: ....

Tongue: ....

Tonsils: ....

Neck: ....

Upper limbs: ....

Chest: ....

Lungs: ....

Heart: ....

Lower limbs: ....

Back: ....

Vital signs: ....

Temperature: ....

Pulse: ....

Respiration: ....

Blood pressure: ....

2. Obstetrical Examination:

   a. Breast Examination:

   Size and shape: ....

   Sensation: ....

   Primary areola: ....

   Secondary areola: ....

   Montgomery tubercles: ....

   Colostrums: ....

   Nipples: ....

   b. Abdominal Examination:

   Inspection: ....

   Size of the abdomen: ....

   Shape of the abdomen: ....

   Contour of the abdominal wall:

   - Skin changes on the abdomen: ....
   - Previous operation scar: ....
   - Striae gravidarum: ....
   - Linea nigra: ....
   - Umbilicus: Flattened/Protruded/Dimpled.

     Visible fetal movement: ....

     Flank region/Filled/Empty

Appearance of the skin infection: ....

Fundal Height (in cm): .... Abdominal girth (in cm): ....

- Abdominal palpation:

Fundal palpation: ....

Lateral palpation: ....

(i) Right lateral palpation: ....

(ii) Left lateral palpation: ....

Pelvic Palpation: ....

Pawlik's grip: ....

Auscultation: ....

- Findings:

Lie: .... Attitude: ....

Presentation: .... Position: ....

Denominator: ....

- Vaginal examination:

Discharge: .... Normal: ....

Abnormal: .... Foul smelling: ....

(VDRL) infection: ....

Investigation done

Date	*Investigation Done*	*Mothers Value*	*Normal Value*	*Remarks*

Any other specific investigation: ....

- Treatment Given: ....

....

....

....

....

Name of the Drug	*Dosag/Route/Frequency*	*Action*	*Side Effects*	*Nurses Responsibility*

Sl No.	*Needs Identified*	*Nursing Care Given*

- Antenatal advices: ....

....

....

....

....

General health condition of the mother: ....

Signature of the Student

Signature of the Supervisor

NURSING CARE PLAN

Assessment	*Nursing Diagnosis*	*Goals*	*Nursing Intervention*	*Rationale*	*Nursing Implementation*	*Evaluation*

NURSING CARE PLAN

Assessment	*Nursing Diagnosis*	*Goals*	*Nursing Intervention*	*Rationale*	*Nursing Implementation*	*Evaluation*

NURSING CARE PLAN

Assessment	*Nursing Diagnosis*	*Goals*	*Nursing Intervention*	*Rationale*	*Nursing Implementation*	*Evaluation*

CHAPTER 3

Normal Deliveries Conducted

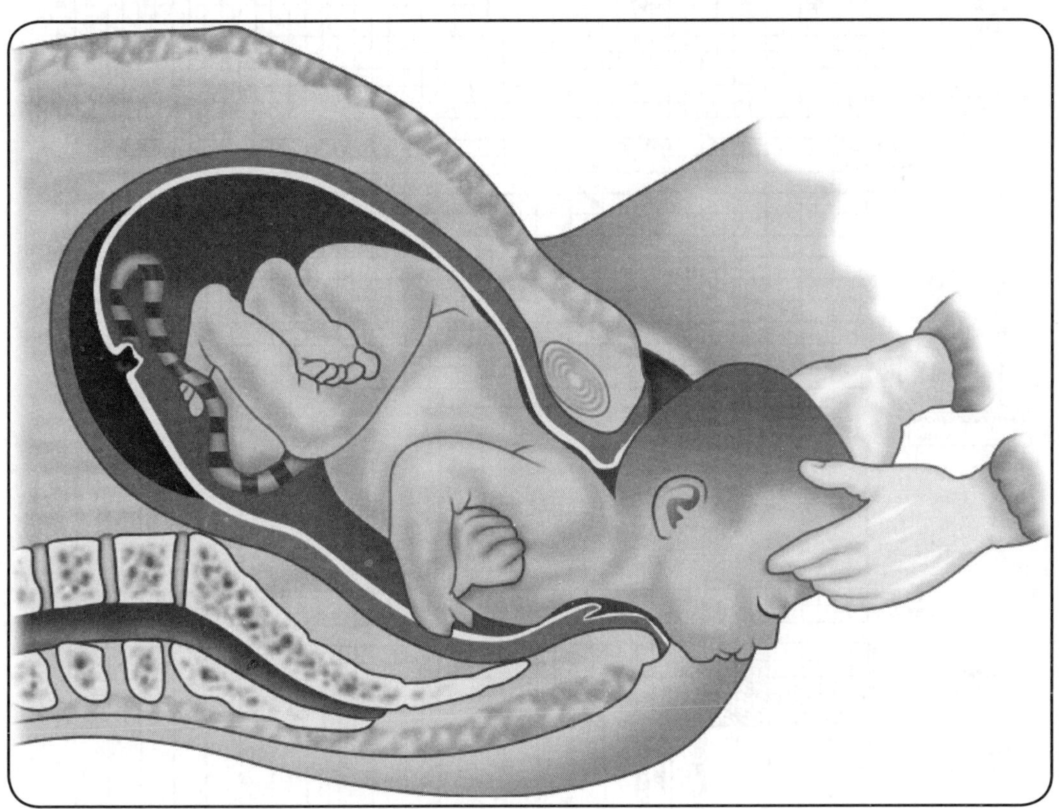

MODEL PARTOGRAPH

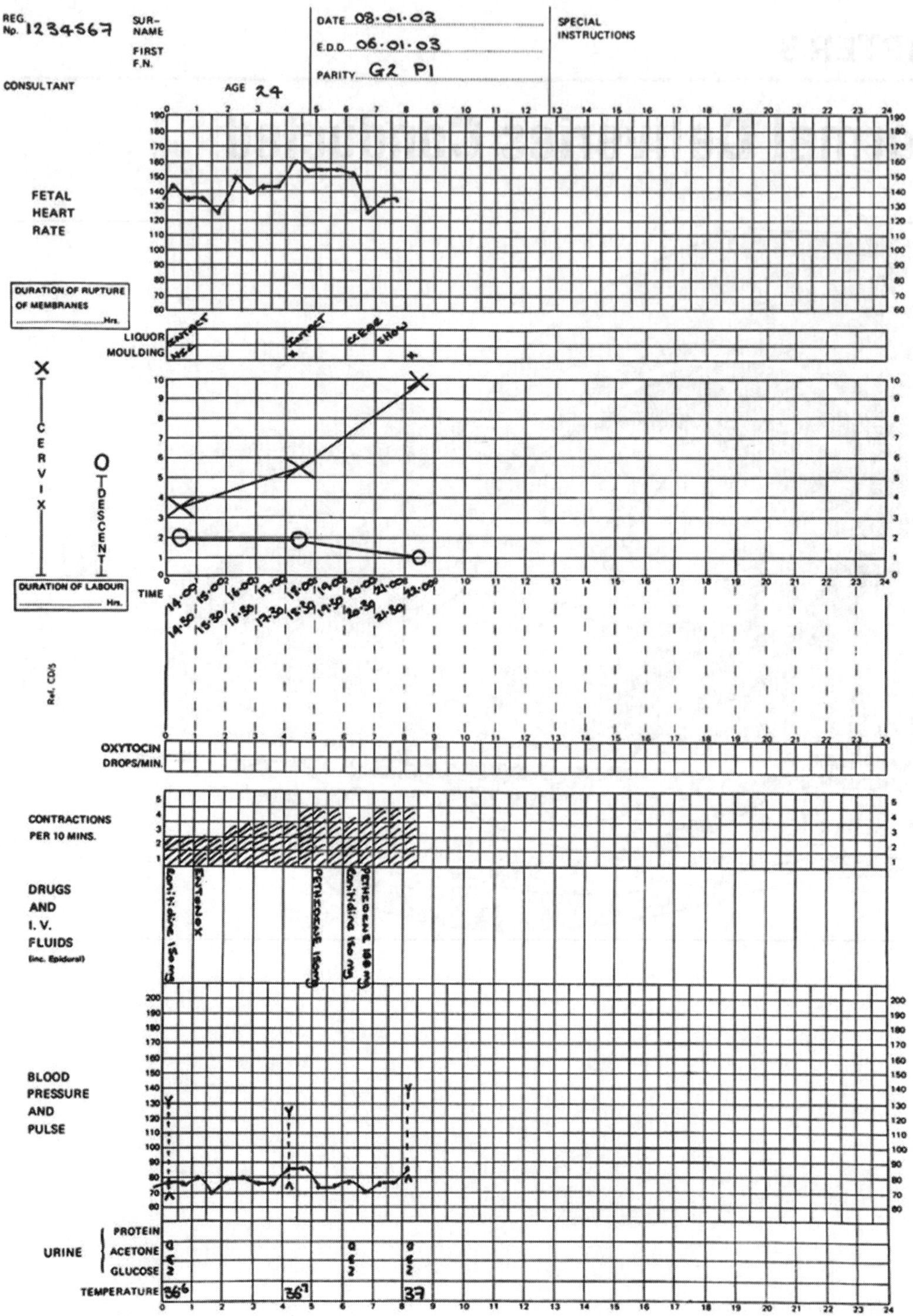

NORMAL DELIVERIES CONDUCTED

Sl No.	IP No.	Name of the Mother	Age	Obstetrical Score	Mode of Delivery	Condition of the Mother			Condition of the Baby			Conducted by
						BP (mm Hg)	Pulse (min)	Height of Fundus (cm)	Weight (kg)	Sex	Apgar Score	
1.												
2.												
3.												
4.												
5.												
6.												
7.												
8.												
9.												

10.												
11.												
12.												
13.												
14.												
15.												
16.												
17.												
18.												
19.												
20.												

NORMAL DELIVERY CONDUCTED (1)

Hospital: ....

Name of the Mother: ....

Age: .... IP No: ....

Date of Admission: .... Date and Time of Delivery: ....

Booked/Unbooked: .... Mode of Delivery: ....

Date of Booking: .... Date of Discharge: ....

Address: ....

Obstetrical score: ....

Last menstrual period (LMP): .... Expected date of delivery (EDD): ....

Educational status:

Husband: .... Wife: ....

Occupation:

Husband: .... Wife: ....

Religion: ....

Labor: 1st stage: .... 2nd stage: .... 3rd stage: ....

ANTENATAL RECORD

Date of Registration: ....

Gestational age at first visit: ....

Sl No.	*Date*	*Weight (kg)*	*Height (cm)*	*Pulse (min)*	*BP (mmHg)*	*Height of Fundus (cm)*	*FHR (mt)*	*Presentation and Position*	*Investigation Done*	*Treatment and Advice Given*

Admission to the Labor Room:

Admission Notes:

- Has been .... hours in labor
- Contraction commenced on .... at ....

- Membranes Intact/Ruptured .... hours ago
- General conditions of the mother: ....

By Palpation:

- Height of the uterus .... weeks
- Condition of the uterus ....
- Position of the fetus ....
- Presentation of the fetus ....
- Abdominal girth ....
- By auscultation ....
- Fetal heart rate (FHR)..

Vaginal Examination:

- Cervical dilation: ....
- Effacement of the cervix: ....
- Station of the head: ....
- Presentation and position: ....
- Membranes ruptured/intact: ....
- Characteristics of the amniotic fluid: ....
- Pelvis: ....

Delivery Notes:

- Membranes ruptured at: ....AM/PM Spontaneously/Artificially
- Os fully dilated at: .... AM/PM
- Expulsive contraction commenced at: .... AM/PM
- Mode of delivery: ....
- Type of episiotomy: ....
- Baby born at: .... AM/PM on: ....
- Sex of the baby: Male/Female
- Weight of the Baby: .... kg
- Condition of the baby when born: Alive/Asphyxiated/Stillbirth
- Apgar score: ....
- Special observation: Cleft Lip/Cleft Palate/Spina Bifida/Talipes
- Suctioning of the oral and nasal route: ....
- Cord ligation: ....
- Meconium passed: ....
- Initiation of breastfeeding: ....

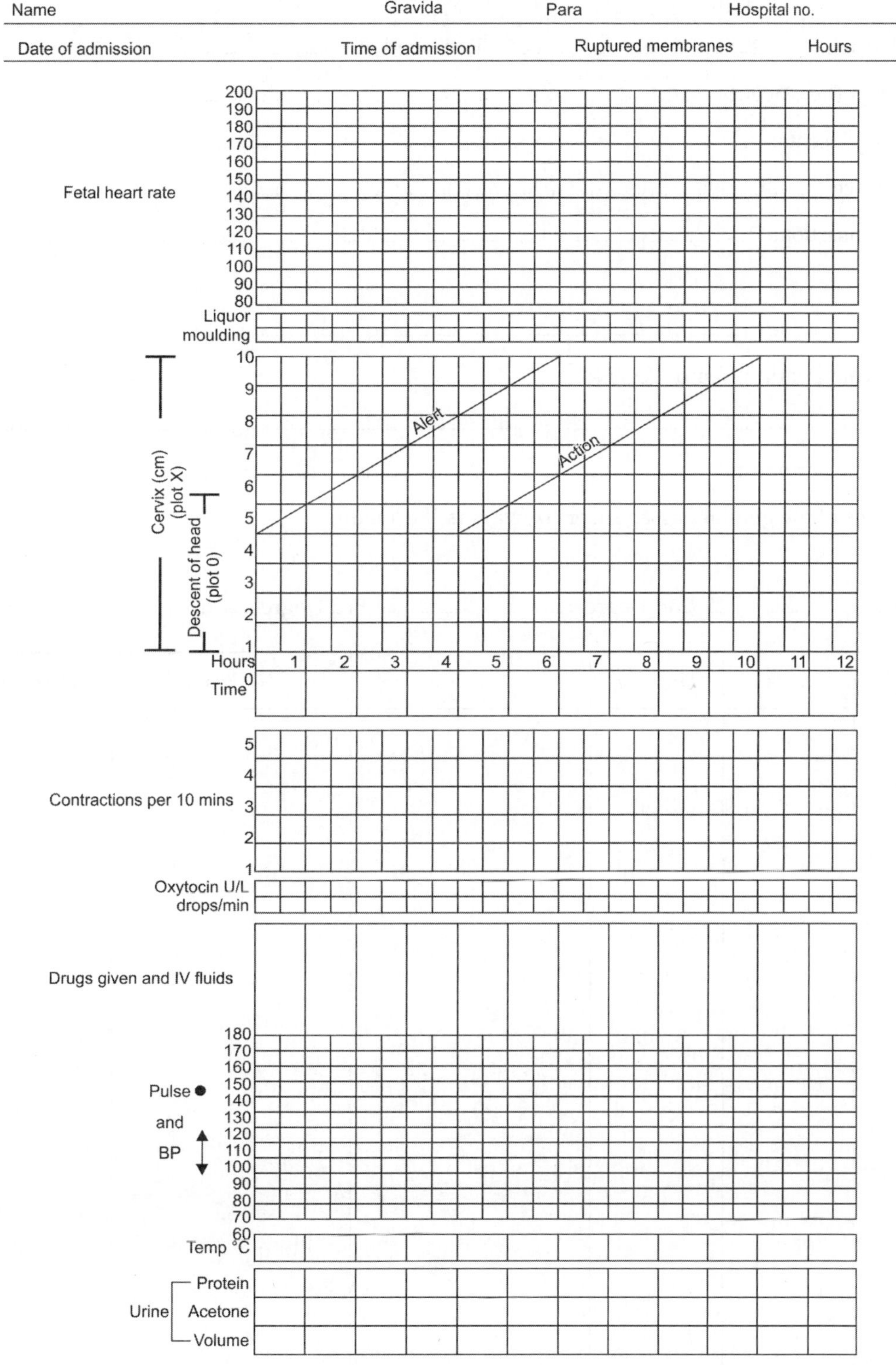
Partograph
Name
Gravida
Para
Hospital no.
Date of admission
Time of admission
Ruptured membranes
Hours
Fetal heart rate
200
190
180
170
160
150
140
130
120
110
100
90
80
Liquor
moulding
Cervix (cm) (plot X)
Descent of head (plot 0)
10
9
8
7
6
5
4
3
2
1
Alert
Action
Hours
1
2
3
4
5
6
7
8
9
10
11
12
Time
0
Contractions per 10 mins
5
4
3
2
1
Oxytocin U/L
drops/min
Drugs given and IV fluids
Pulse ●
and
BP
180
170
160
150
140
130
120
110
100
90
80
70
60
Temp °C
Urine
Protein
Acetone
Volume

DELIVERY OF PLACENTA AND MEMBRANES

- Normal/Manual: .... Removed at: .... AM/PM
- Examination of the placenta: ....
- Weight of the placenta: ....
- Maternal surface: ....
- Type of cord insertion: ....
- Cord length: ....
- Membranes: ....
- Any anatomical variation found: Yes/No
- Specify: ....
- Condition of the perineum: ....
- Any lacerations of the genital passage: Cervix/Vagina/Perineum
- Perineal tear:

  1st Degree: .... 2nd Degree: .... 3rd Degree: .... (Specify if Any)

Drugs Given (name, dosage)	*Route*	*Frequency*	*Action*	*Side Effects*	*Nurses Responsibility*

CONDITION OF THE MOTHER AFTER DELIVERY

Temperature: ....

Pulse: ....

Respiration: ....

Blood pressure: ....

Condition of the neonate: ....

Fundal height: ....

Uterus: ....

Vaginal bleeding: ....

Immediate Care Given:

Needs Identified	*Nursing Care Given*

Conducted by

Assisted by

Signature of the Supervisor

NORMAL DELIVERY CONDUCTED (2)

Hospital: ....

Name of the Mother: ....

Age: .... IP No: ....

Date of Admission: .... Date and Time of Delivery: ....

Booked/Unbooked: .... Mode of Delivery: ....

Date of Booking: .... Date of Discharge: ....

Address: ....

Obstetrical score: ....

Last menstrual period (LMP): .... Expected date of delivery (EDD): ....

Educational status:

Husband: .... Wife: ....

Occupation:

Husband: .... Wife: ....

Religion: ....

Labor: 1st stage: .... 2nd stage: .... 3rd stage: ....

ANTENATAL RECORD

Date of Registration: ....

Gestational age at first visit: ....

Sl No.	*Date*	*Weight (kg)*	*Height (cm)*	*Pulse (min)*	*BP (mmHg)*	*Height of Fundus (cm)*	*FHR (mt)*	*Presentation and Position*	*Investigation Done*	*Treatment and Advice Given*

Admission to the Labor Room:

Admission Notes:

- Has been .... hours in labor
- Contraction commenced on .... at ....

- Membranes Intact/Ruptured .... hours ago
- General conditions of the mother: ....

By Palpation:

- Height of the uterus .... weeks
- Condition of the uterus ....
- Position of the fetus ....
- Presentation of the fetus ....
- Abdominal girth ....
- By auscultation ....
- Fetal heart rate (FHR)..

Vaginal Examination:

- Cervical dilation: ....
- Effacement of the cervix: ....
- Station of the head: ....
- Presentation and position: ....
- Membranes ruptured/intact: ....
- Characteristics of the amniotic fluid: ....
- Pelvis: ....

Delivery Notes:

- Membranes ruptured at: ....AM/PM Spontaneously/Artificially
- Os fully dilated at: .... AM/PM
- Expulsive contraction commenced at: .... AM/PM
- Mode of delivery: ....
- Type of episiotomy: ....
- Baby born at: .... AM/PM on: ....
- Sex of the baby: Male/Female
- Weight of the Baby: .... kg
- Condition of the baby when born: Alive/Asphyxiated/Stillbirth
- Apgar score: ....
- Special observation: Cleft Lip/Cleft Palate/Spina Bifida/Talipes
- Suctioning of the oral and nasal route: ....
- Cord ligation: ....
- Meconium passed: ....
- Initiation of breastfeeding: ....

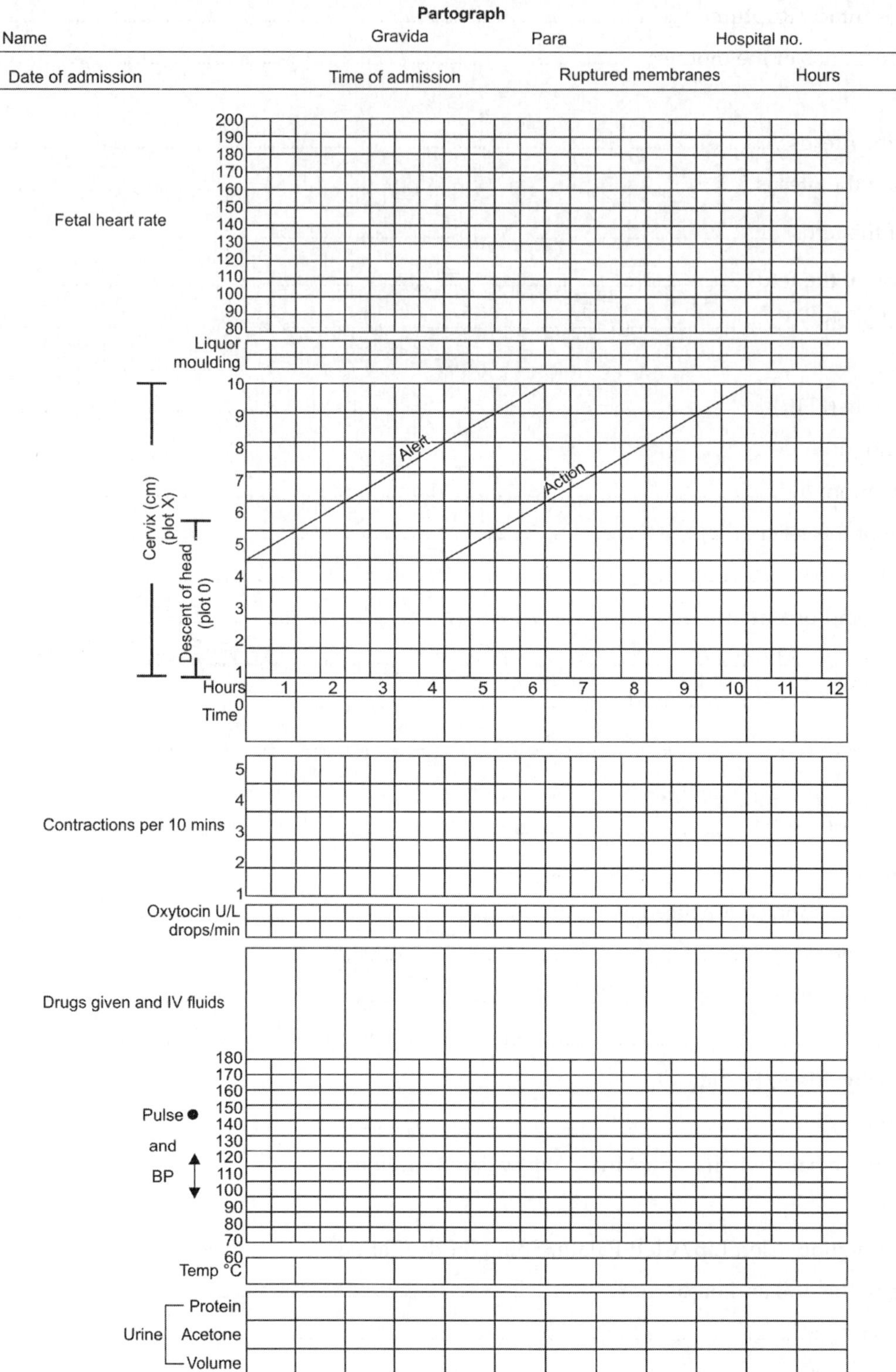
Partograph
Name
Gravida
Para
Hospital no.
Date of admission
Time of admission
Ruptured membranes
Hours
Fetal heart rate
200
190
180
170
160
150
140
130
120
110
100
90
80
Liquor
moulding
Cervix (cm) (plot X)
Descent of head (plot 0)
10
9
8
7
6
5
4
3
2
1
0
Alert
Action
Hours
1
2
3
4
5
6
7
8
9
10
11
12
Time
Contractions per 10 mins
5
4
3
2
1
Oxytocin U/L
drops/min
Drugs given and IV fluids
Pulse ●
and
BP
180
170
160
150
140
130
120
110
100
90
80
70
60
Temp °C
Urine
Protein
Acetone
Volume

DELIVERY OF PLACENTA AND MEMBRANES

- Normal/Manual: .... Removed at: .... AM/PM
- Examination of the placenta: ....
- Weight of the placenta: ....
- Maternal surface: ....
- Type of cord insertion: ....
- Cord length: ....
- Membranes: ....
- Any anatomical variation found: Yes/No
- Specify: ....
- Condition of the perineum: ....
- Any lacerations of the genital passage: Cervix/Vagina/Perineum
- Perineal tear:

  1st Degree: .... 2nd Degree: .... 3rd Degree: .... (Specify if Any)

Drugs Given (name, dosage)	*Route*	*Frequency*	*Action*	*Side Effects*	*Nurses Responsibility*

CONDITION OF THE MOTHER AFTER DELIVERY

Temperature: .... Fundal height: ....

Pulse: .... Uterus: ....

Respiration: .... Vaginal bleeding: ....

Blood pressure: ....

Condition of the neonate: ....

Immediate Care Given:

Needs Identified	*Nursing Care Given*

Conducted by

Assisted by

Signature of the Supervisor

NORMAL DELIVERY CONDUCTED (3)

Hospital: ....

Name of the Mother: ....

Age: .... IP No: ....

Date of Admission: .... Date and Time of Delivery: ....

Booked/Unbooked: .... Mode of Delivery: ....

Date of Booking: .... Date of Discharge: ....

Address: ....

Obstetrical score: ....

Last menstrual period (LMP): .... Expected date of delivery (EDD): ....

Educational status:

Husband: .... Wife: ....

Occupation:

Husband: .... Wife: ....

Religion: ....

Labor: 1st stage: .... 2nd stage: .... 3rd stage: ....

ANTENATAL RECORD

Date of Registration: ....

Gestational age at first visit: ....

Sl No.	*Date*	*Weight (kg)*	*Height (cm)*	*Pulse (min)*	*BP (mmHg)*	*Height of Fundus (cm)*	*FHR (mt)*	*Presentation and Position*	*Investigation Done*	*Treatment and Advice Given*

Admission to the Labor Room:

Admission Notes:

- Has been .... hours in labor
- Contraction commenced on .... at ....

- Membranes Intact/Ruptured .... hours ago
- General conditions of the mother: ....

By Palpation:

- Height of the uterus .... weeks
- Condition of the uterus ....
- Position of the fetus ....
- Presentation of the fetus ....
- Abdominal girth ....
- By auscultation ....
- Fetal heart rate (FHR)..

Vaginal Examination:

- Cervical dilation: ....
- Effacement of the cervix: ....
- Station of the head: ....
- Presentation and position: ....
- Membranes ruptured/intact: ....
- Characteristics of the amniotic fluid: ....
- Pelvis: ....

Delivery Notes:

- Membranes ruptured at: .... AM/PM Spontaneously/Artificially
- Os fully dilated at: .... AM/PM
- Expulsive contraction commenced at: .... AM/PM
- Mode of delivery: ....
- Type of episiotomy: ....
- Baby born at: .... AM/PM on: ....
- Sex of the baby: Male/Female
- Weight of the Baby: .... kg
- Condition of the baby when born: Alive/Asphyxiated/Stillbirth
- Apgar score: ....
- Special observation: Cleft Lip/Cleft Palate/Spina Bifida/Talipes
- Suctioning of the oral and nasal route: ....
- Cord ligation: ....
- Meconium passed: ....
- Initiation of breastfeeding: ....

Partograph

Name | Gravida | Para | Hospital no.

Date of admission | Time of admission | Ruptured membranes | Hours

Fetal heart rate
200 190 180 170 160 150 140 130 120 110 100 90 80

Liquor
moulding

Cervix (cm) (plot X)
Descent of head (plot 0)
10 9 8 7 6 5 4 3 2 1 0

Alert
Action

Hours 1 2 3 4 5 6 7 8 9 10 11 12
Time

Contractions per 10 mins
5 4 3 2 1

Oxytocin U/L
drops/min

Drugs given and IV fluids

Pulse ●
and
BP ↕
180 170 160 150 140 130 120 110 100 90 80 70 60

Temp °C

Urine
Protein
Acetone
Volume

DELIVERY OF PLACENTA AND MEMBRANES

- Normal/Manual: .... Removed at: .... AM/PM
- Examination of the placenta: ....
- Weight of the placenta: ....
- Maternal surface: ....
- Type of cord insertion: ....
- Cord length: ....
- Membranes: ....
- Any anatomical variation found: Yes/No
- Specify: ....
- Condition of the perineum: ....
- Any lacerations of the genital passage: Cervix/Vagina/Perineum
- Perineal tear:

  1st Degree: .... 2nd Degree: .... 3rd Degree: .... (Specify if Any)

Drugs Given (name, dosage)	*Route*	*Frequency*	*Action*	*Side Effects*	*Nurses Responsibility*

CONDITION OF THE MOTHER AFTER DELIVERY

Temperature: ....

Pulse: ....

Respiration: ....

Blood pressure: ....

Condition of the neonate: ....

Fundal height: ....

Uterus: ....

Vaginal bleeding: ....

Immediate Care Given:

Needs Identified	*Nursing Care Given*

Conducted by

Assisted by

Signature of the Supervisor

NORMAL DELIVERY CONDUCTED (4)

Hospital: ....

Name of the Mother: ....

Age: .... IP No: ....

Date of Admission: .... Date and Time of Delivery: ....

Booked/Unbooked: .... Mode of Delivery: ....

Date of Booking: .... Date of Discharge: ....

Address: ....

Obstetrical score: ....

Last menstrual period (LMP): .... Expected date of delivery (EDD): ....

Educational status:

Husband: .... Wife: ....

Occupation:

Husband: .... Wife: ....

Religion: ....

Labor: 1st stage: .... 2nd stage: .... 3rd stage: ....

ANTENATAL RECORD

Date of Registration: ....

Gestational age at first visit: ....

Sl No.	*Date*	*Weight (kg)*	*Height (cm)*	*Pulse (min)*	*BP (mmHg)*	*Height of Fundus (cm)*	*FHR (mt)*	*Presentation and Position*	*Investigation Done*	*Treatment and Advice Given*

Admission to the Labor Room:

Admission Notes:

- Has been .... hours in labor
- Contraction commenced on .... at ....

- Membranes Intact/Ruptured .... hours ago
- General conditions of the mother: ....

By Palpation:

- Height of the uterus .... weeks
- Condition of the uterus ....
- Position of the fetus ....
- Presentation of the fetus ....
- Abdominal girth ....
- By auscultation ....
- Fetal heart rate (FHR)....................

Vaginal Examination:

- Cervical dilation: ....
- Effacement of the cervix: ....
- Station of the head: ....
- Presentation and position: ....
- Membranes ruptured/intact: ....
- Characteristics of the amniotic fluid: ....
- Pelvis: ....

Delivery Notes:

- Membranes ruptured at: ....AM/PM Spontaneously/Artificially
- Os fully dilated at: ....AM/PM
- Expulsive contraction commenced at: ....AM/PM
- Mode of delivery: ....
- Type of episiotomy: ....
- Baby born at: ....AM/PM on: ....
- Sex of the baby: Male/Female
- Weight of the Baby: .... kg
- Condition of the baby when born: Alive/Asphyxiated/Stillbirth
- Apgar score: ....
- Special observation: Cleft Lip/Cleft Palate/Spina Bifida/Talipes
- Suctioning of the oral and nasal route: ....
- Cord ligation: ....
- Meconium passed: ....
- Initiation of breastfeeding: ....

Partograph

Name Gravida Para Hospital no.

Date of admission Time of admission Ruptured membranes Hours

Fetal heart rate

200
190
180
170
160
150
140
130
120
110
100
90
80

Liquor
moulding

Cervix (cm) (plot X)

Descent of head (plot 0)

10
9
8
7
6
5
4
3
2
1

Alert

Action

Hours	1	2	3	4	5	6	7	8	9	10	11	12
Time 0												

Contractions per 10 mins

5
4
3
2
1

Oxytocin U/L
drops/min

Drugs given and IV fluids

Pulse ●

and

BP ↕

180
170
160
150
140
130
120
110
100
90
80
70
60

Temp °C

Urine
- Protein
- Acetone
- Volume

DELIVERY OF PLACENTA AND MEMBRANES

- Normal/Manual: .... Removed at: .... AM/PM
- Examination of the placenta: ....
- Weight of the placenta: ....
- Maternal surface: ....
- Type of cord insertion: ....
- Cord length: ....
- Membranes: ....
- Any anatomical variation found: Yes/No
- Specify: ....
- Condition of the perineum: ....
- Any lacerations of the genital passage: Cervix/Vagina/Perineum
- Perineal tear:

  1st Degree: .... 2nd Degree: .... 3rd Degree: .... (Specify if Any)

Drugs Given (name, dosage)	*Route*	*Frequency*	*Action*	*Side Effects*	*Nurses Responsibility*

CONDITION OF THE MOTHER AFTER DELIVERY

Temperature: ....

Pulse: ....

Respiration: ....

Blood pressure: ....

Condition of the neonate: ....

Fundal height: ....

Uterus: ....

Vaginal bleeding: ....

Immediate Care Given:

Needs Identified	*Nursing Care Given*

Conducted by

Assisted by

Signature of the Supervisor

NORMAL DELIVERY CONDUCTED (5)

Hospital: ....

Name of the Mother: ....

Age: .... IP No: ....

Date of Admission: .... Date and Time of Delivery: ....

Booked/Unbooked: .... Mode of Delivery: ....

Date of Booking: .... Date of Discharge: ....

Address: ....

Obstetrical score: ....

Last menstrual period (LMP): .... Expected date of delivery (EDD): ....

Educational status:

Husband: .... Wife: ....

Occupation:

Husband: .... Wife: ....

Religion: ....

Labor: 1st stage: .... 2nd stage: .... 3rd stage: ....

ANTENATAL RECORD

Date of Registration: ....

Gestational age at first visit: ....

Sl No.	*Date*	*Weight (kg)*	*Height (cm)*	*Pulse (min)*	*BP (mmHg)*	*Height of Fundus (cm)*	*FHR (mt)*	*Presentation and Position*	*Investigation Done*	*Treatment and Advice Given*

Admission to the Labor Room:

Admission Notes:

- Has been .... hours in labor
- Contraction commenced on .... at ....

- Membranes Intact/Ruptured .... hours ago
- General conditions of the mother: ....

By Palpation:

- Height of the uterus .... weeks
- Condition of the uterus ....
- Position of the fetus ....
- Presentation of the fetus ....
- Abdominal girth ....
- By auscultation ....
- Fetal heart rate (FHR)..

Vaginal Examination:

- Cervical dilation: ....
- Effacement of the cervix: ....
- Station of the head: ....
- Presentation and position: ....
- Membranes ruptured/intact: ....
- Characteristics of the amniotic fluid: ....
- Pelvis: ....

Delivery Notes:

- Membranes ruptured at: ....AM/PM Spontaneously/Artificially
- Os fully dilated at: .... AM/PM
- Expulsive contraction commenced at: .... AM/PM
- Mode of delivery: ....
- Type of episiotomy: ....
- Baby born at: .... AM/PM on: ....
- Sex of the baby: Male/Female
- Weight of the Baby: .... kg
- Condition of the baby when born: Alive/Asphyxiated/Stillbirth
- Apgar score: ....
- Special observation: Cleft Lip/Cleft Palate/Spina Bifida/Talipes
- Suctioning of the oral and nasal route: ....
- Cord ligation: ....
- Meconium passed: ....
- Initiation of breastfeeding: ....

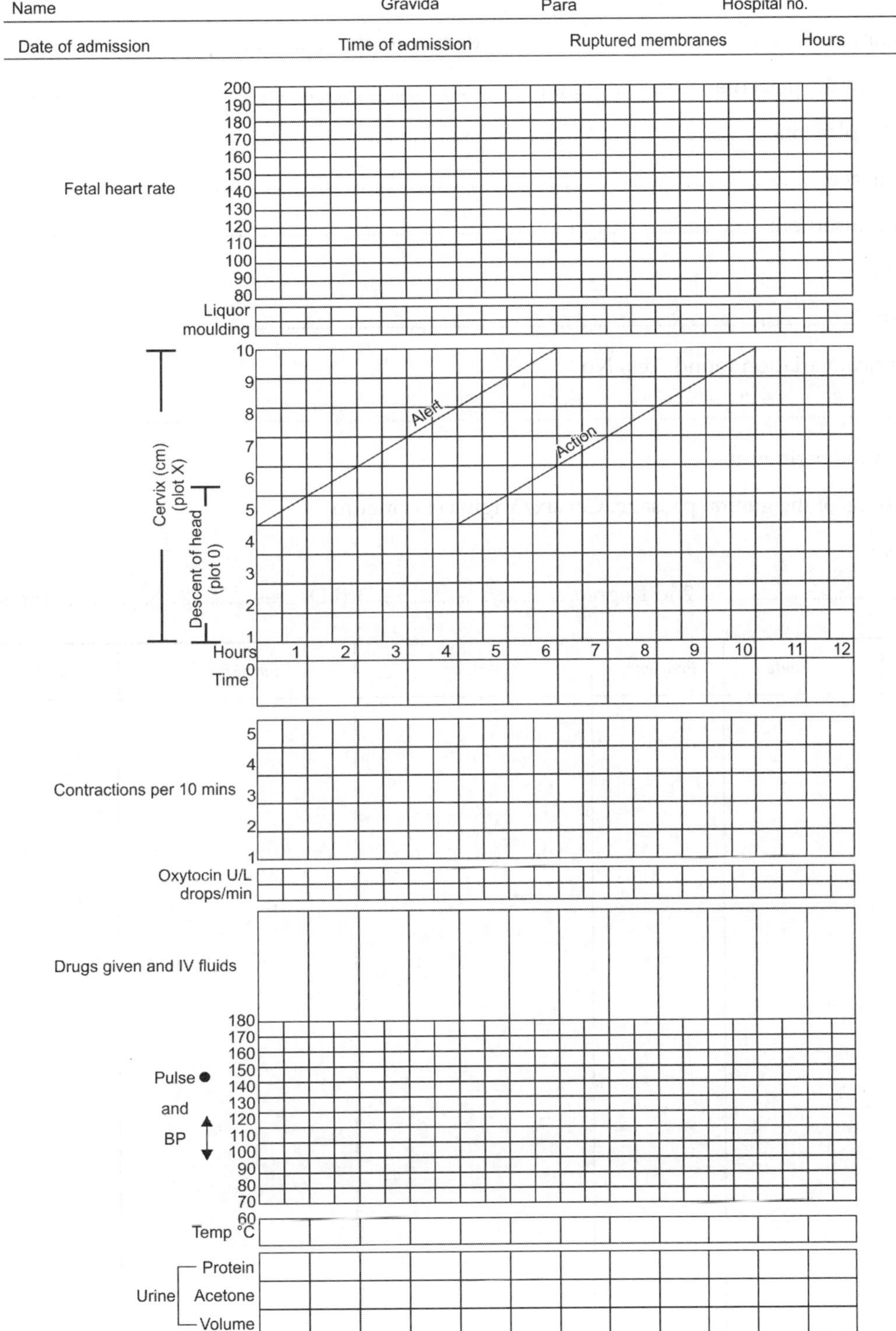
Partograph
Name
Gravida
Para
Hospital no.
Date of admission
Time of admission
Ruptured membranes
Hours
Fetal heart rate
200
190
180
170
160
150
140
130
120
110
100
90
80
Liquor
moulding
Cervix (cm) (plot X)
Descent of head (plot 0)
10
9
8
7
6
5
4
3
2
1
0
Alert
Action
Hours
1
2
3
4
5
6
7
8
9
10
11
12
Time
Contractions per 10 mins
5
4
3
2
1
Oxytocin U/L
drops/min
Drugs given and IV fluids
Pulse ●
and
BP
180
170
160
150
140
130
120
110
100
90
80
70
60
Temp °C
Urine
Protein
Acetone
Volume

DELIVERY OF PLACENTA AND MEMBRANES

- Normal/Manual: .... Removed at: .... AM/PM
- Examination of the placenta: ....
- Weight of the placenta: ....
- Maternal surface: ....
- Type of cord insertion: ....
- Cord length: ....
- Membranes: ....
- Any anatomical variation found: Yes/No
- Specify: ....
- Condition of the perineum: ....
- Any lacerations of the genital passage: Cervix/Vagina/Perineum
- Perineal tear:

  1st Degree: .... 2nd Degree: .... 3rd Degree: .... (Specify if Any)

Drugs Given (name, dosage)	*Route*	*Frequency*	*Action*	*Side Effects*	*Nurses Responsibility*

CONDITION OF THE MOTHER AFTER DELIVERY

Temperature: ....

Pulse: ....

Respiration: ....

Blood pressure: ....

Condition of the neonate: ....

Fundal height: ....

Uterus: ....

Vaginal bleeding: ....

Immediate Care Given:

Needs Identified	*Nursing Care Given*

Conducted by

Assisted by

Signature of the Supervisor

NORMAL DELIVERY CONDUCTED (6)

Hospital: ....

Name of the Mother: ....

Age: .... IP No: ....

Date of Admission: .... Date and Time of Delivery: ....

Booked/Unbooked: .... Mode of Delivery: ....

Date of Booking: .... Date of Discharge: ....

Address: ....

Obstetrical score: ....

Last menstrual period (LMP): .... Expected date of delivery (EDD): ....

Educational status:

Husband: .... Wife: ....

Occupation:

Husband: .... Wife: ....

Religion: ....

Labor: 1st stage: .... 2nd stage: .... 3rd stage: ....

ANTENATAL RECORD

Date of Registration: ....

Gestational age at first visit: ....

Sl No.	*Date*	*Weight (kg)*	*Height (cm)*	*Pulse (min)*	*BP (mmHg)*	*Height of Fundus (cm)*	*FHR (mt)*	*Presentation and Position*	*Investigation Done*	*Treatment and Advice Given*

Admission to the Labor Room:

Admission Notes:

- Has been .... hours in labor
- Contraction commenced on .... at ....

- Membranes Intact/Ruptured .... hours ago
- General conditions of the mother: ....

By Palpation:

- Height of the uterus .... weeks
- Condition of the uterus ....
- Position of the fetus ....
- Presentation of the fetus ....
- Abdominal girth ....
- By auscultation ....
- Fetal heart rate (FHR)..

Vaginal Examination:

- Cervical dilation: ....
- Effacement of the cervix: ....
- Station of the head: ....
- Presentation and position: ....
- Membranes ruptured/intact: ....
- Characteristics of the amniotic fluid: ....
- Pelvis: ....

Delivery Notes:

- Membranes ruptured at: .... AM/PM Spontaneously/Artificially
- Os fully dilated at: .... AM/PM
- Expulsive contraction commenced at: .... AM/PM
- Mode of delivery: ....
- Type of episiotomy: ....
- Baby born at: .... AM/PM on: ....
- Sex of the baby: Male/Female
- Weight of the Baby: .... kg
- Condition of the baby when born: Alive/Asphyxiated/Stillbirth
- Apgar score: ....
- Special observation: Cleft Lip/Cleft Palate/Spina Bifida/Talipes
- Suctioning of the oral and nasal route: ....
- Cord ligation: ....
- Meconium passed: ....
- Initiation of breastfeeding: ....

Partograph

Name Gravida Para Hospital no.

Date of admission Time of admission Ruptured membranes Hours

Fetal heart rate

200
190
180
170
160
150
140
130
120
110
100
90
80

Liquor
moulding

Cervix (cm) (plot X)

Descent of head (plot 0)

10
9
8
7
6
5
4
3
2
1

Alert

Action

Hours	1	2	3	4	5	6	7	8	9	10	11	12
0 Time												

Contractions per 10 mins

5
4
3
2
1

Oxytocin U/L
drops/min

Drugs given and IV fluids

Pulse ●

and

BP ↕

180
170
160
150
140
130
120
110
100
90
80
70
60

Temp °C

Urine
- Protein
- Acetone
- Volume

DELIVERY OF PLACENTA AND MEMBRANES

- Normal/Manual: .... Removed at: .... AM/PM
- Examination of the placenta: ....
- Weight of the placenta: ....
- Maternal surface: ....
- Type of cord insertion: ....
- Cord length: ....
- Membranes: ....
- Any anatomical variation found: Yes/No
- Specify: ....
- Condition of the perineum: ....
- Any lacerations of the genital passage: Cervix/Vagina/Perineum
- Perineal tear:

  1st Degree: .... 2nd Degree: .... 3rd Degree: .... (Specify if Any)

Drugs Given (name, dosage)	*Route*	*Frequency*	*Action*	*Side Effects*	*Nurses Responsibility*

CONDITION OF THE MOTHER AFTER DELIVERY

Temperature: ....

Pulse: ....

Respiration: ....

Blood pressure: ....

Condition of the neonate: ....

Fundal height: ....

Uterus: ....

Vaginal bleeding: ....

Immediate Care Given:

Needs Identified	*Nursing Care Given*

Conducted by

Assisted by

Signature of the Supervisor

NORMAL DELIVERY CONDUCTED (7)

Hospital: ....

Name of the Mother: ....

Age: .... IP No: ....

Date of Admission: .... Date and Time of Delivery: ....

Booked/Unbooked: .... Mode of Delivery: ....

Date of Booking: .... Date of Discharge: ....

Address: ....

Obstetrical score: ....

Last menstrual period (LMP): .... Expected date of delivery (EDD): ....

Educational status:

Husband: .... Wife: ....

Occupation:

Husband: .... Wife: ....

Religion: ....

Labor: 1st stage: .... 2nd stage: .... 3rd stage: ....

ANTENATAL RECORD

Date of Registration: ....

Gestational age at first visit: ....

Sl No.	*Date*	*Weight (kg)*	*Height (cm)*	*Pulse (min)*	*BP (mmHg)*	*Height of Fundus (cm)*	*FHR (mt)*	*Presentation and Position*	*Investigation Done*	*Treatment and Advice Given*

Admission to the Labor Room:

Admission Notes:

- Has been .... hours in labor
- Contraction commenced on .... at ....

- Membranes Intact/Ruptured .... hours ago
- General conditions of the mother: ....

By Palpation:

- Height of the uterus .... weeks
- Condition of the uterus ....
- Position of the fetus ....
- Presentation of the fetus ....
- Abdominal girth ....
- By auscultation ....
- Fetal heart rate (FHR)..

Vaginal Examination:

- Cervical dilation: ....
- Effacement of the cervix: ....
- Station of the head: ....
- Presentation and position: ....
- Membranes ruptured/intact: ....
- Characteristics of the amniotic fluid: ....
- Pelvis: ....

Delivery Notes:

- Membranes ruptured at: .... AM/PM Spontaneously/Artificially
- Os fully dilated at: .... AM/PM
- Expulsive contraction commenced at: .... AM/PM
- Mode of delivery: ....
- Type of episiotomy: ....
- Baby born at: .... AM/PM on: ....
- Sex of the baby: Male/Female
- Weight of the Baby: .... kg
- Condition of the baby when born: Alive/Asphyxiated/Stillbirth
- Apgar score: ....
- Special observation: Cleft Lip/Cleft Palate/Spina Bifida/Talipes
- Suctioning of the oral and nasal route: ....
- Cord ligation: ....
- Meconium passed: ....
- Initiation of breastfeeding: ....

Partograph

Name Gravida Para Hospital no.

Date of admission Time of admission Ruptured membranes Hours

Fetal heart rate
200 190 180 170 160 150 140 130 120 110 100 90 80

Liquor
moulding

Cervix (cm) (plot X)
Descent of head (plot 0)
10 9 8 7 6 5 4 3 2 1 0

Alert
Action

Hours 1 2 3 4 5 6 7 8 9 10 11 12
Time

Contractions per 10 mins
5 4 3 2 1

Oxytocin U/L
drops/min

Drugs given and IV fluids

Pulse ●
and
BP ↕
180 170 160 150 140 130 120 110 100 90 80 70 60

Temp °C

Urine
- Protein
- Acetone
- Volume

DELIVERY OF PLACENTA AND MEMBRANES

- Normal/Manual: .... Removed at: .... AM/PM
- Examination of the placenta: ....
- Weight of the placenta: ....
- Maternal surface: ....
- Type of cord insertion: ....
- Cord length: ....
- Membranes: ....
- Any anatomical variation found: Yes/No
- Specify: ....
- Condition of the perineum: ....
- Any lacerations of the genital passage: Cervix/Vagina/Perineum
- Perineal tear:

  1st Degree: .... 2nd Degree: .... 3rd Degree: .... (Specify if Any)

Drugs Given (name, dosage)	*Route*	*Frequency*	*Action*	*Side Effects*	*Nurses Responsibility*

CONDITION OF THE MOTHER AFTER DELIVERY

Temperature: ....

Pulse: ....

Respiration: ....

Blood pressure: ....

Condition of the neonate: ....

Fundal height: ....

Uterus: ....

Vaginal bleeding: ....

Immediate Care Given:

Needs Identified	*Nursing Care Given*

Conducted by

Assisted by

Signature of the Supervisor

NORMAL DELIVERY CONDUCTED (8)

Hospital: ....

Name of the Mother: ....

Age: .... IP No: ....

Date of Admission: .... Date and Time of Delivery: ....

Booked/Unbooked: .... Mode of Delivery: ....

Date of Booking: .... Date of Discharge: ....

Address: ....

Obstetrical score: ....

Last menstrual period (LMP): .... Expected date of delivery (EDD): ....

Educational status:

Husband: .... Wife: ....

Occupation:

Husband: .... Wife: ....

Religion: ....

Labor: 1st stage: .... 2nd stage: .... 3rd stage: ....

ANTENATAL RECORD

Date of Registration: ....

Gestational age at first visit: ....

Sl No.	*Date*	*Weight (kg)*	*Height (cm)*	*Pulse (min)*	*BP (mmHg)*	*Height of Fundus (cm)*	*FHR (mt)*	*Presentation and Position*	*Investigation Done*	*Treatment and Advice Given*

Admission to the Labor Room:

Admission Notes:

- Has been .... hours in labor
- Contraction commenced on .... at ....

- Membranes Intact/Ruptured .... hours ago
- General conditions of the mother: ....

By Palpation:

- Height of the uterus .... weeks
- Condition of the uterus ....
- Position of the fetus ....
- Presentation of the fetus ....
- Abdominal girth ....
- By auscultation ....
- Fetal heart rate (FHR)..

Vaginal Examination:

- Cervical dilation: ....
- Effacement of the cervix: ....
- Station of the head: ....
- Presentation and position: ....
- Membranes ruptured/intact: ....
- Characteristics of the amniotic fluid: ....
- Pelvis: ....

Delivery Notes:

- Membranes ruptured at: .... AM/PM Spontaneously/Artificially
- Os fully dilated at: .... AM/PM
- Expulsive contraction commenced at: .... AM/PM
- Mode of delivery: ....
- Type of episiotomy: ....
- Baby born at: .... AM/PM on: ....
- Sex of the baby: Male/Female
- Weight of the Baby: .... kg
- Condition of the baby when born: Alive/Asphyxiated/Stillbirth
- Apgar score: ....
- Special observation: Cleft Lip/Cleft Palate/Spina Bifida/Talipes
- Suctioning of the oral and nasal route: ....
- Cord ligation: ....
- Meconium passed: ....
- Initiation of breastfeeding: ....

Partograph

Name Gravida Para Hospital no.

Date of admission Time of admission Ruptured membranes Hours

Fetal heart rate

200 190 180 170 160 150 140 130 120 110 100 90 80

Liquor

moulding

Cervix (cm) (plot X)

Descent of head (plot 0)

10 9 8 7 6 5 4 3 2 1 0

Alert

Action

Hours	1	2	3	4	5	6	7	8	9	10	11	12
Time												

Contractions per 10 mins

5 4 3 2 1

Oxytocin U/L

drops/min

Drugs given and IV fluids

Pulse ●

and

BP ↕

180 170 160 150 140 130 120 110 100 90 80 70 60

Temp °C

Urine

- Protein
- Acetone
- Volume

DELIVERY OF PLACENTA AND MEMBRANES

- Normal/Manual: .... Removed at: .... AM/PM
- Examination of the placenta: ....
- Weight of the placenta: ....
- Maternal surface: ....
- Type of cord insertion: ....
- Cord length: ....
- Membranes: ....
- Any anatomical variation found: Yes/No
- Specify: ....
- Condition of the perineum: ....
- Any lacerations of the genital passage: Cervix/Vagina/Perineum
- Perineal tear:

  1st Degree: .... 2nd Degree: .... 3rd Degree: .... (Specify if Any)

Drugs Given (name, dosage)	*Route*	*Frequency*	*Action*	*Side Effects*	*Nurses Responsibility*

CONDITION OF THE MOTHER AFTER DELIVERY

Temperature: ....

Pulse: ....

Respiration: ....

Blood pressure: ....

Condition of the neonate: ....

Fundal height: ....

Uterus: ....

Vaginal bleeding: ....

Immediate Care Given:

Needs Identified	*Nursing Care Given*

Conducted by

Assisted by

Signature of the Supervisor

NORMAL DELIVERY CONDUCTED (9)

Hospital: ....

Name of the Mother: ....

Age: .... IP No: ....

Date of Admission: .... Date and Time of Delivery: ....

Booked/Unbooked: .... Mode of Delivery: ....

Date of Booking: .... Date of Discharge: ....

Address: ....

Obstetrical score: ....

Last menstrual period (LMP): .... Expected date of delivery (EDD): ....

Educational status:

Husband: .... Wife: ....

Occupation:

Husband: .... Wife: ....

Religion: ....

Labor: 1st stage: .... 2nd stage: .... 3rd stage: ....

ANTENATAL RECORD

Date of Registration: ....

Gestational age at first visit: ....

Sl No.	*Date*	*Weight (kg)*	*Height (cm)*	*Pulse (min)*	*BP (mmHg)*	*Height of Fundus (cm)*	*FHR (mt)*	*Presentation and Position*	*Investigation Done*	*Treatment and Advice Given*

Admission to the Labor Room:

Admission Notes:

- Has been .... hours in labor
- Contraction commenced on .... at ....

- Membranes Intact/Ruptured .... hours ago
- General conditions of the mother: ....

By Palpation:

- Height of the uterus .... weeks
- Condition of the uterus ....
- Position of the fetus ....
- Presentation of the fetus ....
- Abdominal girth ....
- By auscultation ....
- Fetal heart rate (FHR)....................

Vaginal Examination:

- Cervical dilation: ....
- Effacement of the cervix: ....
- Station of the head: ....
- Presentation and position: ....
- Membranes ruptured/intact: ....
- Characteristics of the amniotic fluid: ....
- Pelvis: ....

Delivery Notes:

- Membranes ruptured at: .... AM/PM Spontaneously/Artificially
- Os fully dilated at: .... AM/PM
- Expulsive contraction commenced at: .... AM/PM
- Mode of delivery: ....
- Type of episiotomy: ....
- Baby born at: .... AM/PM on: ....
- Sex of the baby: Male/Female
- Weight of the Baby: .... kg
- Condition of the baby when born: Alive/Asphyxiated/Stillbirth
- Apgar score: ....
- Special observation: Cleft Lip/Cleft Palate/Spina Bifida/Talipes
- Suctioning of the oral and nasal route: ....
- Cord ligation: ....
- Meconium passed: ....
- Initiation of breastfeeding: ....

Partograph

Name Gravida Para Hospital no.

Date of admission Time of admission Ruptured membranes Hours

Fetal heart rate
200
190
180
170
160
150
140
130
120
110
100
90
80

Liquor
moulding

Cervix (cm) (plot X)
Descent of head (plot 0)
10
9
8
7
6
5
4
3
2
1
0

Alert
Action

Hours	1	2	3	4	5	6	7	8	9	10	11	12
Time												

Contractions per 10 mins
5
4
3
2
1

Oxytocin U/L
drops/min

Drugs given and IV fluids

Pulse ●
and
BP ↕
180
170
160
150
140
130
120
110
100
90
80
70
60

Temp °C

Urine
Protein
Acetone
Volume

DELIVERY OF PLACENTA AND MEMBRANES

- Normal/Manual: .... Removed at: .... AM/PM
- Examination of the placenta: ....
- Weight of the placenta: ....
- Maternal surface: ....
- Type of cord insertion: ....
- Cord length: ....
- Membranes: ....
- Any anatomical variation found: Yes/No
- Specify: ....
- Condition of the perineum: ....
- Any lacerations of the genital passage: Cervix/Vagina/Perineum
- Perineal tear:

  1st Degree: .... 2nd Degree: .... 3rd Degree: .... (Specify if Any)

Drugs Given (name, dosage)	*Route*	*Frequency*	*Action*	*Side Effects*	*Nurses Responsibility*

CONDITION OF THE MOTHER AFTER DELIVERY

Temperature: ....

Fundal height: ....

Pulse: ....

Uterus: ....

Respiration: ....

Vaginal bleeding: ....

Blood pressure: ....

Condition of the neonate: ....

Immediate Care Given:

Needs Identified	*Nursing Care Given*

Conducted by

Assisted by

Signature of the Supervisor

NORMAL DELIVERY CONDUCTED (10)

Hospital: ....

Name of the Mother: ....

Age: .... IP No: ....

Date of Admission: .... Date and Time of Delivery: ....

Booked/Unbooked: .... Mode of Delivery: ....

Date of Booking: .... Date of Discharge: ....

Address: ....

Obstetrical score: ....

Last menstrual period (LMP): .... Expected date of delivery (EDD): ....

Educational status:

Husband: .... Wife: ....

Occupation:

Husband: .... Wife: ....

Religion: ....

Labor: 1st stage: .... 2nd stage: .... 3rd stage: ....

ANTENATAL RECORD

Date of Registration: ....

Gestational age at first visit: ....

Sl No.	*Date*	*Weight (kg)*	*Height (cm)*	*Pulse (min)*	*BP (mmHg)*	*Height of Fundus (cm)*	*FHR (mt)*	*Presentation and Position*	*Investigation Done*	*Treatment and Advice Given*

Admission to the Labor Room:

Admission Notes:

- Has been .... hours in labor
- Contraction commenced on .... at ....

- Membranes Intact/Ruptured .... hours ago
- General conditions of the mother: ....

By Palpation:

- Height of the uterus .... weeks
- Condition of the uterus ....
- Position of the fetus ....
- Presentation of the fetus ....
- Abdominal girth ....
- By auscultation ....
- Fetal heart rate (FHR)....................

Vaginal Examination:

- Cervical dilation: ....
- Effacement of the cervix: ....
- Station of the head: ....
- Presentation and position: ....
- Membranes ruptured/intact: ....
- Characteristics of the amniotic fluid: ....
- Pelvis: ....

Delivery Notes:

- Membranes ruptured at: .... AM/PM Spontaneously/Artificially
- Os fully dilated at: .... AM/PM
- Expulsive contraction commenced at: .... AM/PM
- Mode of delivery: ....
- Type of episiotomy: ....
- Baby born at: .... AM/PM on: ....
- Sex of the baby: Male/Female
- Weight of the Baby: .... kg
- Condition of the baby when born: Alive/Asphyxiated/Stillbirth
- Apgar score: ....
- Special observation: Cleft Lip/Cleft Palate/Spina Bifida/Talipes
- Suctioning of the oral and nasal route: ....
- Cord ligation: ....
- Meconium passed: ....
- Initiation of breastfeeding: ....

Partograph

Name Gravida Para Hospital no.

Date of admission Time of admission Ruptured membranes Hours

DELIVERY OF PLACENTA AND MEMBRANES

- Normal/Manual: .... Removed at: .... AM/PM
- Examination of the placenta: ....
- Weight of the placenta: ....
- Maternal surface: ....
- Type of cord insertion: ....
- Cord length: ....
- Membranes: ....
- Any anatomical variation found: Yes/No
- Specify: ....
- Condition of the perineum: ....
- Any lacerations of the genital passage: Cervix/Vagina/Perineum
- Perineal tear:

  1st Degree: .... 2nd Degree: .... 3rd Degree: .... (Specify if Any)

Drugs Given (name, dosage)	*Route*	*Frequency*	*Action*	*Side Effects*	*Nurses Responsibility*

CONDITION OF THE MOTHER AFTER DELIVERY

Temperature: ....

Pulse: ....

Respiration: ....

Blood pressure: ....

Condition of the neonate: ....

Fundal height: ....

Uterus: ....

Vaginal bleeding: ....

Immediate Care Given:

Needs Identified	*Nursing Care Given*

Conducted by

Assisted by

Signature of the Supervisor

NORMAL DELIVERY CONDUCTED (11)

Hospital: ....

Name of the Mother: ....

Age: .... IP No: ....

Date of Admission: .... Date and Time of Delivery: ....

Booked/Unbooked: .... Mode of Delivery: ....

Date of Booking: .... Date of Discharge: ....

Address: ....

Obstetrical score: ....

Last menstrual period (LMP): .... Expected date of delivery (EDD): ....

Educational status:

Husband: .... Wife: ....

Occupation:

Husband: .... Wife: ....

Religion: ....

Labor: 1st stage: .... 2nd stage: .... 3rd stage: ....

ANTENATAL RECORD

Date of Registration: ....

Gestational age at first visit: ....

Sl No.	*Date*	*Weight (kg)*	*Height (cm)*	*Pulse (min)*	*BP (mmHg)*	*Height of Fundus (cm)*	*FHR (mt)*	*Presentation and Position*	*Investigation Done*	*Treatment and Advice Given*

Admission to the Labor Room:

Admission Notes:

- Has been .... hours in labor
- Contraction commenced on .... at ....

- Membranes Intact/Ruptured .... hours ago
- General conditions of the mother: ....

By Palpation:

- Height of the uterus .... weeks
- Condition of the uterus ....
- Position of the fetus ....
- Presentation of the fetus ....
- Abdominal girth ....
- By auscultation ....
- Fetal heart rate (FHR)..

Vaginal Examination:

- Cervical dilation: ....
- Effacement of the cervix: ....
- Station of the head: ....
- Presentation and position: ....
- Membranes ruptured/intact: ....
- Characteristics of the amniotic fluid: ....
- Pelvis: ....

Delivery Notes:

- Membranes ruptured at: .... AM/PM Spontaneously/Artificially
- Os fully dilated at: .... AM/PM
- Expulsive contraction commenced at: .... AM/PM
- Mode of delivery: ....
- Type of episiotomy: ....
- Baby born at: .... AM/PM on: ....
- Sex of the baby: Male/Female
- Weight of the Baby: .... kg
- Condition of the baby when born: Alive/Asphyxiated/Stillbirth
- Apgar score: ....
- Special observation: Cleft Lip/Cleft Palate/Spina Bifida/Talipes
- Suctioning of the oral and nasal route: ....
- Cord ligation: ....
- Meconium passed: ....
- Initiation of breastfeeding: ....

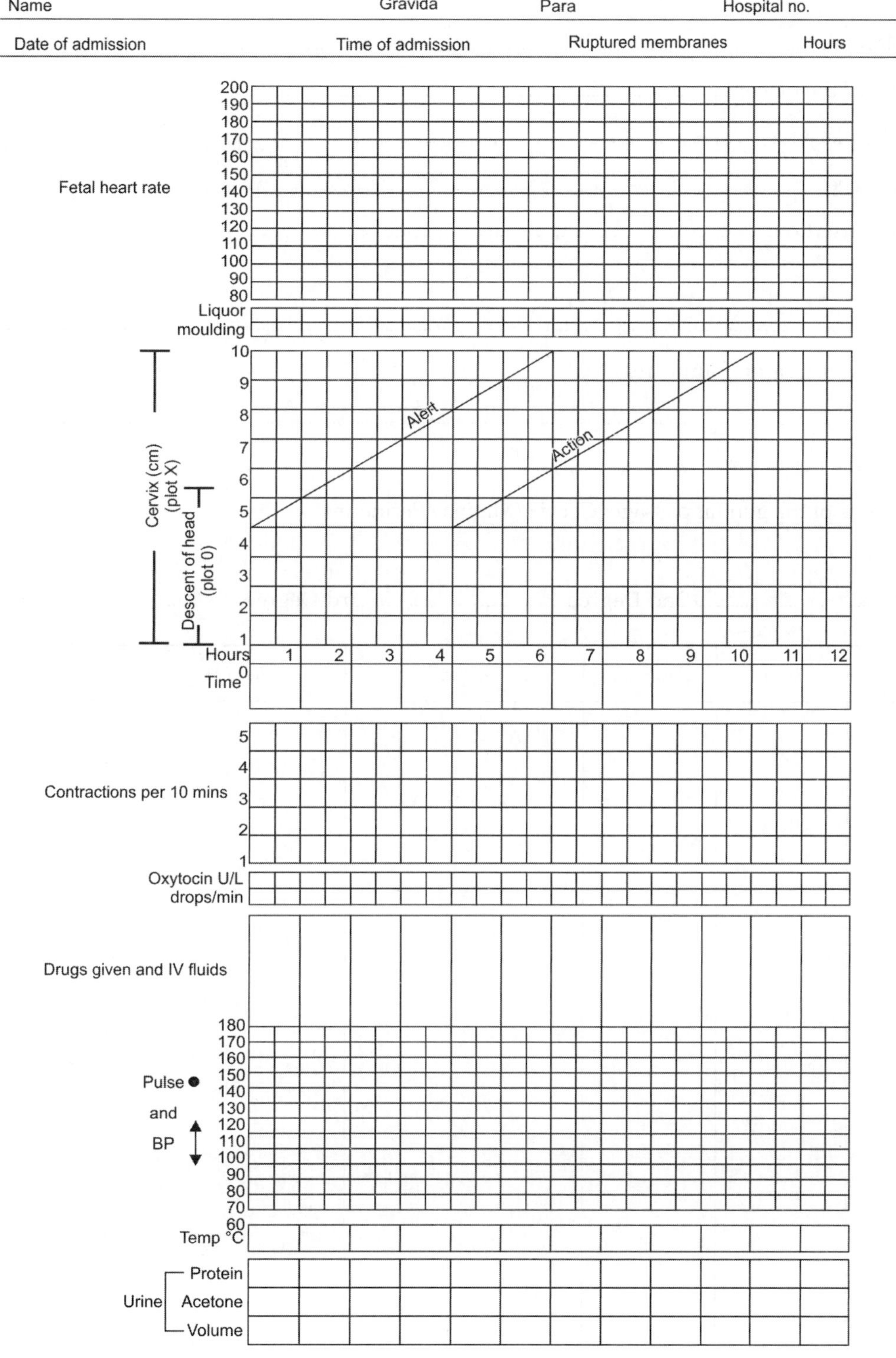
Partograph
Name
Gravida
Para
Hospital no.
Date of admission
Time of admission
Ruptured membranes
Hours
Fetal heart rate
200
190
180
170
160
150
140
130
120
110
100
90
80
Liquor
moulding
Cervix (cm) (plot X)
Descent of head (plot 0)
10
9
8
7
6
5
4
3
2
1
0
Alert
Action
Hours
1
2
3
4
5
6
7
8
9
10
11
12
Time
Contractions per 10 mins
5
4
3
2
1
Oxytocin U/L
drops/min
Drugs given and IV fluids
Pulse ●
and
BP
180
170
160
150
140
130
120
110
100
90
80
70
60
Temp °C
Urine
Protein
Acetone
Volume

DELIVERY OF PLACENTA AND MEMBRANES

- Normal/Manual: .... Removed at: .... AM/PM
- Examination of the placenta: ....
- Weight of the placenta: ....
- Maternal surface: ....
- Type of cord insertion: ....
- Cord length: ....
- Membranes: ....
- Any anatomical variation found: Yes/No
- Specify: ....
- Condition of the perineum: ....
- Any lacerations of the genital passage: Cervix/Vagina/Perineum
- Perineal tear:

  1st Degree: .... 2nd Degree: .... 3rd Degree: .... (Specify if Any)

Drugs Given (name, dosage)	*Route*	*Frequency*	*Action*	*Side Effects*	*Nurses Responsibility*

CONDITION OF THE MOTHER AFTER DELIVERY

Temperature: .... Fundal height: ....

Pulse: .... Uterus: ....

Respiration: .... Vaginal bleeding: ....

Blood pressure: ....

Condition of the neonate: ....

Immediate Care Given:

Needs Identified	*Nursing Care Given*

Conducted by

Assisted by

Signature of the Supervisor

NORMAL DELIVERY CONDUCTED (12)

Hospital: ....

Name of the Mother: ....

Age: .... IP No: ....

Date of Admission: .... Date and Time of Delivery: ....

Booked/Unbooked: .... Mode of Delivery: ....

Date of Booking: .... Date of Discharge: ....

Address: ....

Obstetrical score: ....

Last menstrual period (LMP): .... Expected date of delivery (EDD): ....

Educational status:

Husband: .... Wife: ....

Occupation:

Husband: .... Wife: ....

Religion: ....

Labor: 1st stage: .... 2nd stage: .... 3rd stage: ....

ANTENATAL RECORD

Date of Registration: ....

Gestational age at first visit: ....

Sl No.	*Date*	*Weight (kg)*	*Height (cm)*	*Pulse (min)*	*BP (mmHg)*	*Height of Fundus (cm)*	*FHR (mt)*	*Presentation and Position*	*Investigation Done*	*Treatment and Advice Given*

Admission to the Labor Room:

Admission Notes:

- Has been .... hours in labor
- Contraction commenced on .... at ....

- Membranes Intact/Ruptured .... hours ago
- General conditions of the mother: ....

By Palpation:

- Height of the uterus .... weeks
- Condition of the uterus ....
- Position of the fetus ....
- Presentation of the fetus ....
- Abdominal girth ....
- By auscultation ....
- Fetal heart rate (FHR)..

Vaginal Examination:

- Cervical dilation: ....
- Effacement of the cervix: ....
- Station of the head: ....
- Presentation and position: ....
- Membranes ruptured/intact: ....
- Characteristics of the amniotic fluid: ....
- Pelvis: ....

Delivery Notes:

- Membranes ruptured at: ....AM/PM Spontaneously/Artificially
- Os fully dilated at: .... AM/PM
- Expulsive contraction commenced at: .... AM/PM
- Mode of delivery: ....
- Type of episiotomy: ....
- Baby born at: .... AM/PM on: ....
- Sex of the baby: Male/Female
- Weight of the Baby: .... kg
- Condition of the baby when born: Alive/Asphyxiated/Stillbirth
- Apgar score: ....
- Special observation: Cleft Lip/Cleft Palate/Spina Bifida/Talipes
- Suctioning of the oral and nasal route: ....
- Cord ligation: ....
- Meconium passed: ....
- Initiation of breastfeeding: ....

Partograph

Name Gravida Para Hospital no.

Date of admission Time of admission Ruptured membranes Hours

Fetal heart rate 200 190 180 170 160 150 140 130 120 110 100 90 80

Liquor

moulding

Cervix (cm) (plot X)

Descent of head (plot 0)

10 9 8 7 6 5 4 3 2 1 0

Alert

Action

Hours	1	2	3	4	5	6	7	8	9	10	11	12
Time												

Contractions per 10 mins 5 4 3 2 1

Oxytocin U/L

drops/min

Drugs given and IV fluids

Pulse ● and BP ↕ 180 170 160 150 140 130 120 110 100 90 80 70 60

Temp °C

Urine: Protein, Acetone, Volume

DELIVERY OF PLACENTA AND MEMBRANES

- Normal/Manual: .... Removed at: .... AM/PM
- Examination of the placenta: ....
- Weight of the placenta: ....
- Maternal surface: ....
- Type of cord insertion: ....
- Cord length: ....
- Membranes: ....
- Any anatomical variation found: Yes/No
- Specify: ....
- Condition of the perineum: ....
- Any lacerations of the genital passage: Cervix/Vagina/Perineum
- Perineal tear:

  1st Degree: .... 2nd Degree: .... 3rd Degree: .... (Specify if Any)

Drugs Given (name, dosage)	*Route*	*Frequency*	*Action*	*Side Effects*	*Nurses Responsibility*

CONDITION OF THE MOTHER AFTER DELIVERY

Temperature: ....

Fundal height: ....

Pulse: ....

Uterus: ....

Respiration: ....

Vaginal bleeding: ....

Blood pressure: ....

Condition of the neonate: ....

Immediate Care Given:

Needs Identified	*Nursing Care Given*

Conducted by

Assisted by

Signature of the Supervisor

NORMAL DELIVERY CONDUCTED (13)

Hospital: ....

Name of the Mother: ....

Age: .... IP No: ....

Date of Admission: .... Date and Time of Delivery: ....

Booked/Unbooked: .... Mode of Delivery: ....

Date of Booking: .... Date of Discharge: ....

Address: ....

Obstetrical score: ....

Last menstrual period (LMP): .... Expected date of delivery (EDD): ....

Educational status:

Husband: .... Wife: ....

Occupation:

Husband: .... Wife: ....

Religion: ....

Labor: 1st stage: .... 2nd stage: .... 3rd stage: ....

ANTENATAL RECORD

Date of Registration: ....

Gestational age at first visit: ....

Sl No.	*Date*	*Weight (kg)*	*Height (cm)*	*Pulse (min)*	*BP (mmHg)*	*Height of Fundus (cm)*	*FHR (mt)*	*Presentation and Position*	*Investigation Done*	*Treatment and Advice Given*

Admission to the Labor Room:

Admission Notes:

- Has been .... hours in labor
- Contraction commenced on .... at ....

- Membranes Intact/Ruptured .... hours ago
- General conditions of the mother: ....

By Palpation:

- Height of the uterus .... weeks
- Condition of the uterus ....
- Position of the fetus ....
- Presentation of the fetus ....
- Abdominal girth ....
- By auscultation ....
- Fetal heart rate (FHR)..

Vaginal Examination:

- Cervical dilation: ....
- Effacement of the cervix: ....
- Station of the head: ....
- Presentation and position: ....
- Membranes ruptured/intact: ....
- Characteristics of the amniotic fluid: ....
- Pelvis: ....

Delivery Notes:

- Membranes ruptured at: ....AM/PM Spontaneously/Artificially
- Os fully dilated at: ....AM/PM
- Expulsive contraction commenced at: ....AM/PM
- Mode of delivery: ....
- Type of episiotomy: ....
- Baby born at: .... AM/PM on: ....
- Sex of the baby: Male/Female
- Weight of the Baby: .... kg
- Condition of the baby when born: Alive/Asphyxiated/Stillbirth
- Apgar score: ....
- Special observation: Cleft Lip/Cleft Palate/Spina Bifida/Talipes
- Suctioning of the oral and nasal route: ....
- Cord ligation: ....
- Meconium passed: ....
- Initiation of breastfeeding: ....

Partograph

Name Gravida Para Hospital no.

Date of admission Time of admission Ruptured membranes Hours

Fetal heart rate: 200, 190, 180, 170, 160, 150, 140, 130, 120, 110, 100, 90, 80

Liquor

moulding

Cervix (cm) (plot X)

Descent of head (plot 0)

10, 9, 8, 7, 6, 5, 4, 3, 2, 1, 0

Alert

Action

Hours: 1, 2, 3, 4, 5, 6, 7, 8, 9, 10, 11, 12

Time

Contractions per 10 mins: 5, 4, 3, 2, 1

Oxytocin U/L

drops/min

Drugs given and IV fluids

Pulse ●

and

BP ↕

180, 170, 160, 150, 140, 130, 120, 110, 100, 90, 80, 70, 60

Temp °C

Urine: Protein, Acetone, Volume

DELIVERY OF PLACENTA AND MEMBRANES

- Normal/Manual: .... Removed at: .... AM/PM
- Examination of the placenta: ....
- Weight of the placenta: ....
- Maternal surface: ....
- Type of cord insertion: ....
- Cord length: ....
- Membranes: ....
- Any anatomical variation found: Yes/No
- Specify: ....
- Condition of the perineum: ....
- Any lacerations of the genital passage: Cervix/Vagina/Perineum
- Perineal tear:

  1st Degree: .... 2nd Degree: .... 3rd Degree: .... (Specify if Any)

Drugs Given (name, dosage)	*Route*	*Frequency*	*Action*	*Side Effects*	*Nurses Responsibility*

CONDITION OF THE MOTHER AFTER DELIVERY

Temperature: ....

Pulse: ....

Respiration: ....

Blood pressure: ....

Condition of the neonate: ....

Fundal height: ....

Uterus: ....

Vaginal bleeding: ....

Immediate Care Given:

Needs Identified	*Nursing Care Given*

Conducted by

Assisted by

Signature of the Supervisor

NORMAL DELIVERY CONDUCTED (14)

Hospital: ....

Name of the Mother: ....

Age: .... IP No: ....

Date of Admission: .... Date and Time of Delivery: ....

Booked/Unbooked: .... Mode of Delivery: ....

Date of Booking: .... Date of Discharge: ....

Address: ....

Obstetrical score: ....

Last menstrual period (LMP): .... Expected date of delivery (EDD): ....

Educational status:

Husband: .... Wife: ....

Occupation:

Husband: .... Wife: ....

Religion: ....

Labor: 1st stage: .... 2nd stage: .... 3rd stage: ....

ANTENATAL RECORD

Date of Registration: ....

Gestational age at first visit: ....

Sl No.	*Date*	*Weight (kg)*	*Height (cm)*	*Pulse (min)*	*BP (mmHg)*	*Height of Fundus (cm)*	*FHR (mt)*	*Presentation and Position*	*Investigation Done*	*Treatment and Advice Given*

Admission to the Labor Room:

Admission Notes:

- Has been .... hours in labor
- Contraction commenced on .... at ....

- Membranes Intact/Ruptured .... hours ago
- General conditions of the mother: ....

By Palpation:

- Height of the uterus .... weeks
- Condition of the uterus ....
- Position of the fetus ....
- Presentation of the fetus ....
- Abdominal girth ....
- By auscultation ....
- Fetal heart rate (FHR)..

Vaginal Examination:

- Cervical dilation: ....
- Effacement of the cervix: ....
- Station of the head: ....
- Presentation and position: ....
- Membranes ruptured/intact: ....
- Characteristics of the amniotic fluid: ....
- Pelvis: ....

Delivery Notes:

- Membranes ruptured at: .... AM/PM Spontaneously/Artificially
- Os fully dilated at: .... AM/PM
- Expulsive contraction commenced at: .... AM/PM
- Mode of delivery: ....
- Type of episiotomy: ....
- Baby born at: .... AM/PM on: ....
- Sex of the baby: Male/Female
- Weight of the Baby: .... kg
- Condition of the baby when born: Alive/Asphyxiated/Stillbirth
- Apgar score: ....
- Special observation: Cleft Lip/Cleft Palate/Spina Bifida/Talipes
- Suctioning of the oral and nasal route: ....
- Cord ligation: ....
- Meconium passed: ....
- Initiation of breastfeeding: ....

Partograph

Name | Gravida | Para | Hospital no.

Date of admission | Time of admission | Ruptured membranes | Hours

Fetal heart rate: 200, 190, 180, 170, 160, 150, 140, 130, 120, 110, 100, 90, 80

Liquor
moulding

Cervix (cm) (plot X)
Descent of head (plot 0)
10, 9, 8, 7, 6, 5, 4, 3, 2, 1, 0

Alert
Action

Hours: 1, 2, 3, 4, 5, 6, 7, 8, 9, 10, 11, 12

Time

Contractions per 10 mins: 5, 4, 3, 2, 1

Oxytocin U/L
drops/min

Drugs given and IV fluids

Pulse ●
and
BP ↕
180, 170, 160, 150, 140, 130, 120, 110, 100, 90, 80, 70, 60

Temp °C

Urine: Protein, Acetone, Volume

DELIVERY OF PLACENTA AND MEMBRANES

- Normal/Manual: .... Removed at: .... AM/PM
- Examination of the placenta: ....
- Weight of the placenta: ....
- Maternal surface: ....
- Type of cord insertion: ....
- Cord length: ....
- Membranes: ....
- Any anatomical variation found: Yes/No
- Specify: ....
- Condition of the perineum: ....
- Any lacerations of the genital passage: Cervix/Vagina/Perineum
- Perineal tear:

  1st Degree: .... 2nd Degree: .... 3rd Degree: .... (Specify if Any)

Drugs Given (name, dosage)	*Route*	*Frequency*	*Action*	*Side Effects*	*Nurses Responsibility*

CONDITION OF THE MOTHER AFTER DELIVERY

Temperature: ....

Pulse: ....

Respiration: ....

Blood pressure: ....

Condition of the neonate: ....

Fundal height: ....

Uterus: ....

Vaginal bleeding: ....

Immediate Care Given:

Needs Identified	*Nursing Care Given*

Conducted by

Assisted by

Signature of the Supervisor

NORMAL DELIVERY CONDUCTED (15)

Hospital: ....

Name of the Mother: ....

Age: .... IP No: ....

Date of Admission: .... Date and Time of Delivery: ....

Booked/Unbooked: .... Mode of Delivery: ....

Date of Booking: .... Date of Discharge: ....

Address: ....

Obstetrical score: ....

Last menstrual period (LMP): .... Expected date of delivery (EDD): ....

Educational status:

Husband: .... Wife: ....

Occupation:

Husband: .... Wife: ....

Religion: ....

Labor: 1st stage: .... 2nd stage: .... 3rd stage: ....

ANTENATAL RECORD

Date of Registration: ....

Gestational age at first visit: ....

Sl No.	*Date*	*Weight (kg)*	*Height (cm)*	*Pulse (min)*	*BP (mmHg)*	*Height of Fundus (cm)*	*FHR (mt)*	*Presentation and Position*	*Investigation Done*	*Treatment and Advice Given*

Admission to the Labor Room:

Admission Notes:

- Has been .... hours in labor
- Contraction commenced on .... at ....

- Membranes Intact/Ruptured .... hours ago
- General conditions of the mother: ....

By Palpation:

- Height of the uterus .... weeks
- Condition of the uterus ....
- Position of the fetus ....
- Presentation of the fetus ....
- Abdominal girth ....
- By auscultation ....
- Fetal heart rate (FHR)..

Vaginal Examination:

- Cervical dilation: ....
- Effacement of the cervix: ....
- Station of the head: ....
- Presentation and position: ....
- Membranes ruptured/intact: ....
- Characteristics of the amniotic fluid: ....
- Pelvis: ....

Delivery Notes:

- Membranes ruptured at: ....AM/PM Spontaneously/Artificially
- Os fully dilated at: ....AM/PM
- Expulsive contraction commenced at: ....AM/PM
- Mode of delivery: ....
- Type of episiotomy: ....
- Baby born at: .... AM/PM on: ....
- Sex of the baby: Male/Female
- Weight of the Baby: .... kg
- Condition of the baby when born: Alive/Asphyxiated/Stillbirth
- Apgar score: ....
- Special observation: Cleft Lip/Cleft Palate/Spina Bifida/Talipes
- Suctioning of the oral and nasal route: ....
- Cord ligation: ....
- Meconium passed: ....
- Initiation of breastfeeding: ....

Partograph

Name Gravida Para Hospital no.

Date of admission Time of admission Ruptured membranes Hours

Fetal heart rate

200 190 180 170 160 150 140 130 120 110 100 90 80

Liquor
moulding

Cervix (cm) (plot X)

Descent of head (plot 0)

10 9 8 7 6 5 4 3 2 1

Alert

Action

Hours	1	2	3	4	5	6	7	8	9	10	11	12
Time 0												

Contractions per 10 mins

5 4 3 2 1

Oxytocin U/L
drops/min

Drugs given and IV fluids

Pulse ●
and
BP ↕

180 170 160 150 140 130 120 110 100 90 80 70 60

Temp °C

Urine
- Protein
- Acetone
- Volume

DELIVERY OF PLACENTA AND MEMBRANES

- Normal/Manual: .... Removed at: .... AM/PM
- Examination of the placenta: ....
- Weight of the placenta: ....
- Maternal surface: ....
- Type of cord insertion: ....
- Cord length: ....
- Membranes: ....
- Any anatomical variation found: Yes/No
- Specify: ....
- Condition of the perineum: ....
- Any lacerations of the genital passage: Cervix/Vagina/Perineum
- Perineal tear:

  1st Degree: .... 2nd Degree: .... 3rd Degree: .... (Specify if Any)

Drugs Given (name, dosage)	*Route*	*Frequency*	*Action*	*Side Effects*	*Nurses Responsibility*

CONDITION OF THE MOTHER AFTER DELIVERY

Temperature: ....

Pulse: ....

Respiration: ....

Blood pressure: ....

Condition of the neonate: ....

Fundal height: ....

Uterus: ....

Vaginal bleeding: ....

Immediate Care Given:

Needs Identified	*Nursing Care Given*

Conducted by

Assisted by

Signature of the Supervisor

NORMAL DELIVERY CONDUCTED (16)

Hospital: ....

Name of the Mother: ....

Age: .... IP No: ....

Date of Admission: .... Date and Time of Delivery: ....

Booked/Unbooked: .... Mode of Delivery: ....

Date of Booking: .... Date of Discharge: ....

Address: ....

Obstetrical score: ....

Last menstrual period (LMP): .... Expected date of delivery (EDD): ....

Educational status:

Husband: .... Wife: ....

Occupation:

Husband: .... Wife: ....

Religion: ....

Labor: 1st stage: .... 2nd stage: .... 3rd stage: ....

ANTENATAL RECORD

Date of Registration: ....

Gestational age at first visit: ....

Sl No.	*Date*	*Weight (kg)*	*Height (cm)*	*Pulse (min)*	*BP (mmHg)*	*Height of Fundus (cm)*	*FHR (mt)*	*Presentation and Position*	*Investigation Done*	*Treatment and Advice Given*

Admission to the Labor Room:

Admission Notes:

- Has been .... hours in labor
- Contraction commenced on .... at ....

- Membranes Intact/Ruptured .... hours ago
- General conditions of the mother: ....

By Palpation:

- Height of the uterus .... weeks
- Condition of the uterus ....
- Position of the fetus ....
- Presentation of the fetus ....
- Abdominal girth ....
- By auscultation ....
- Fetal heart rate (FHR)....................

Vaginal Examination:

- Cervical dilation: ....
- Effacement of the cervix: ....
- Station of the head: ....
- Presentation and position: ....
- Membranes ruptured/intact: ....
- Characteristics of the amniotic fluid: ....
- Pelvis: ....

Delivery Notes:

- Membranes ruptured at: .... AM/PM Spontaneously/Artificially
- Os fully dilated at: .... AM/PM
- Expulsive contraction commenced at: .... AM/PM
- Mode of delivery: ....
- Type of episiotomy: ....
- Baby born at: .... AM/PM on: ....
- Sex of the baby: Male/Female
- Weight of the Baby: .... kg
- Condition of the baby when born: Alive/Asphyxiated/Stillbirth
- Apgar score: ....
- Special observation: Cleft Lip/Cleft Palate/Spina Bifida/Talipes
- Suctioning of the oral and nasal route: ....
- Cord ligation: ....
- Meconium passed: ....
- Initiation of breastfeeding: ....

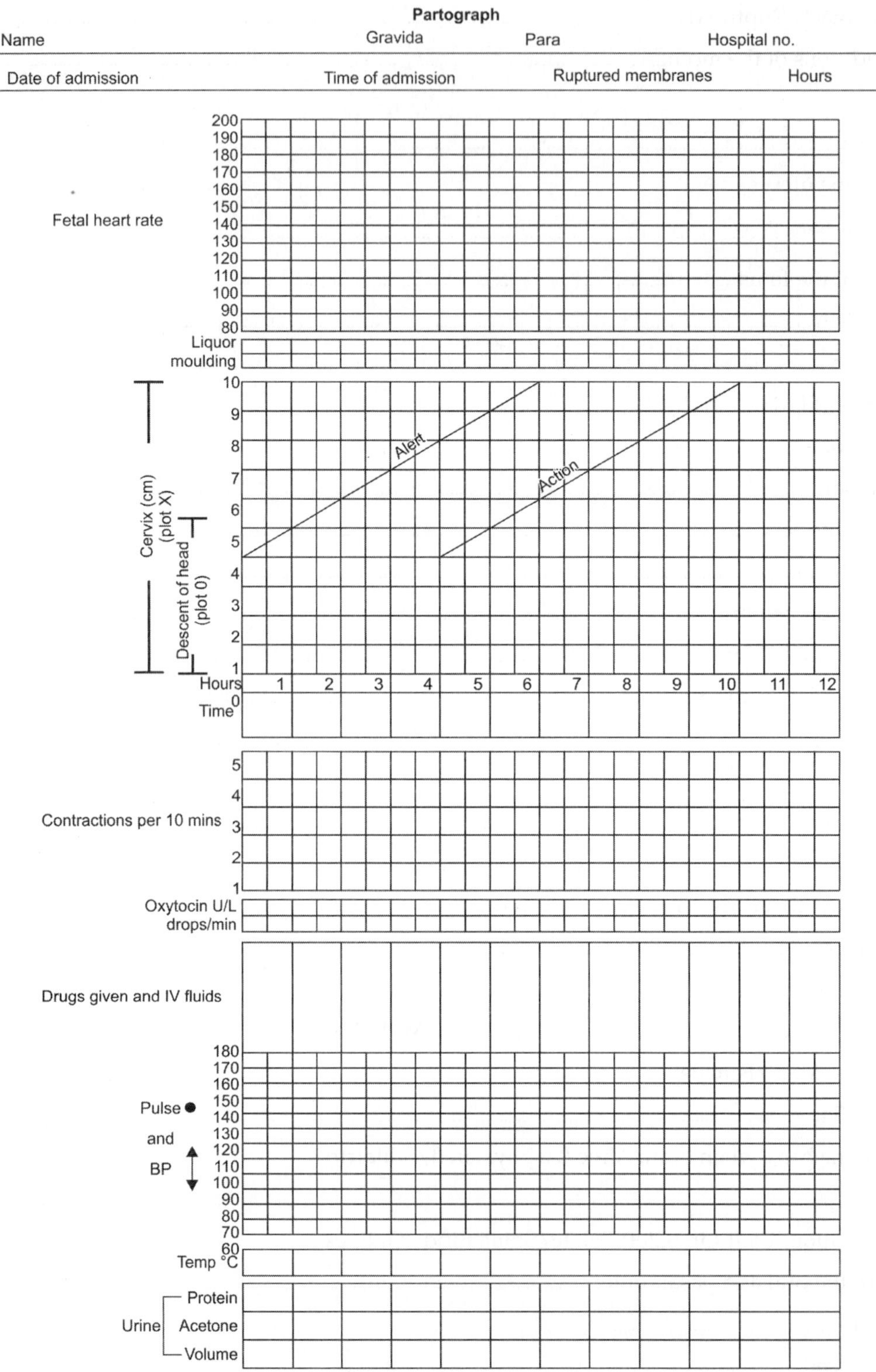
Partograph
Name
Gravida
Para
Hospital no.
Date of admission
Time of admission
Ruptured membranes
Hours
Fetal heart rate
200
190
180
170
160
150
140
130
120
110
100
90
80
Liquor
moulding
Cervix (cm) (plot X)
Descent of head (plot 0)
10
9
8
7
6
5
4
3
2
1
0
Alert
Action
Hours
1 2 3 4 5 6 7 8 9 10 11 12
Time
Contractions per 10 mins
5
4
3
2
1
Oxytocin U/L
drops/min
Drugs given and IV fluids
Pulse ●
and
BP
180
170
160
150
140
130
120
110
100
90
80
70
60
Temp °C
Urine
Protein
Acetone
Volume

DELIVERY OF PLACENTA AND MEMBRANES

- Normal/Manual: .... Removed at: .... AM/PM
- Examination of the placenta: ....
- Weight of the placenta: ....
- Maternal surface: ....
- Type of cord insertion: ....
- Cord length: ....
- Membranes: ....
- Any anatomical variation found: Yes/No
- Specify: ....
- Condition of the perineum: ....
- Any lacerations of the genital passage: Cervix/Vagina/Perineum
- Perineal tear:

  1st Degree: .... 2nd Degree: .... 3rd Degree: .... (Specify if Any)

Drugs Given (name, dosage)	*Route*	*Frequency*	*Action*	*Side Effects*	*Nurses Responsibility*

CONDITION OF THE MOTHER AFTER DELIVERY

Temperature: ....

Pulse: ....

Respiration: ....

Blood pressure: ....

Condition of the neonate: ....

Fundal height: ....

Uterus: ....

Vaginal bleeding: ....

Immediate Care Given:

Needs Identified	*Nursing Care Given*

Conducted by

Assisted by

Signature of the Supervisor

NORMAL DELIVERY CONDUCTED (17)

Hospital: ....

Name of the Mother: ....

Age: .... IP No: ....

Date of Admission: .... Date and Time of Delivery: ....

Booked/Unbooked: .... Mode of Delivery: ....

Date of Booking: .... Date of Discharge: ....

Address: ....

Obstetrical score: ....

Last menstrual period (LMP): .... Expected date of delivery (EDD): ....

Educational status:

Husband: .... Wife: ....

Occupation:

Husband: .... Wife: ....

Religion: ....

Labor: 1st stage: .... 2nd stage: .... 3rd stage: ....

ANTENATAL RECORD

Date of Registration: ....

Gestational age at first visit: ....

Sl No.	*Date*	*Weight (kg)*	*Height (cm)*	*Pulse (min)*	*BP (mmHg)*	*Height of Fundus (cm)*	*FHR (mt)*	*Presentation and Position*	*Investigation Done*	*Treatment and Advice Given*

Admission to the Labor Room:

Admission Notes:

- Has been .... hours in labor
- Contraction commenced on .... at ....

- Membranes Intact/Ruptured .... hours ago
- General conditions of the mother: ....

By Palpation:

- Height of the uterus .... weeks
- Condition of the uterus ....
- Position of the fetus ....
- Presentation of the fetus ....
- Abdominal girth ....
- By auscultation ....
- Fetal heart rate (FHR)............

Vaginal Examination:

- Cervical dilation: ....
- Effacement of the cervix: ....
- Station of the head: ....
- Presentation and position: ....
- Membranes ruptured/intact: ....
- Characteristics of the amniotic fluid: ....
- Pelvis: ....

Delivery Notes:

- Membranes ruptured at: .... AM/PM Spontaneously/Artificially
- Os fully dilated at: .... AM/PM
- Expulsive contraction commenced at: .... AM/PM
- Mode of delivery: ....
- Type of episiotomy: ....
- Baby born at: .... AM/PM on: ....
- Sex of the baby: Male/Female
- Weight of the Baby: .... kg
- Condition of the baby when born: Alive/Asphyxiated/Stillbirth
- Apgar score: ....
- Special observation: Cleft Lip/Cleft Palate/Spina Bifida/Talipes
- Suctioning of the oral and nasal route: ....
- Cord ligation: ....
- Meconium passed: ....
- Initiation of breastfeeding: ....

Partograph

Name Gravida Para Hospital no.

Date of admission Time of admission Ruptured membranes Hours

Fetal heart rate: 200, 190, 180, 170, 160, 150, 140, 130, 120, 110, 100, 90, 80

Liquor
moulding

Cervix (cm) (plot X)
Descent of head (plot 0)

10, 9, 8, 7, 6, 5, 4, 3, 2, 1

Alert

Action

Hours	1	2	3	4	5	6	7	8	9	10	11	12
0 Time												

Contractions per 10 mins: 5, 4, 3, 2, 1

Oxytocin U/L
drops/min

Drugs given and IV fluids

Pulse ●
and
BP ↕

180, 170, 160, 150, 140, 130, 120, 110, 100, 90, 80, 70, 60

Temp °C

Urine	
	Protein
	Acetone
	Volume

DELIVERY OF PLACENTA AND MEMBRANES

- Normal/Manual: .... Removed at: .... AM/PM
- Examination of the placenta: ....
- Weight of the placenta: ....
- Maternal surface: ....
- Type of cord insertion: ....
- Cord length: ....
- Membranes: ....
- Any anatomical variation found: Yes/No
- Specify: ....
- Condition of the perineum: ....
- Any lacerations of the genital passage: Cervix/Vagina/Perineum
- Perineal tear:

  1st Degree: .... 2nd Degree: .... 3rd Degree: .... (Specify if Any)

Drugs Given (name, dosage)	*Route*	*Frequency*	*Action*	*Side Effects*	*Nurses Responsibility*

CONDITION OF THE MOTHER AFTER DELIVERY

Temperature: ....

Fundal height: ....

Pulse: ....

Uterus: ....

Respiration: ....

Vaginal bleeding: ....

Blood pressure: ....

Condition of the neonate: ....

Immediate Care Given:

Needs Identified	*Nursing Care Given*

Conducted by

Assisted by

Signature of the Supervisor

NORMAL DELIVERY CONDUCTED (18)

Hospital: ....

Name of the Mother: ....

Age: .... IP No: ....

Date of Admission: .... Date and Time of Delivery: ....

Booked/Unbooked: .... Mode of Delivery: ....

Date of Booking: .... Date of Discharge: ....

Address: ....

Obstetrical score: ....

Last menstrual period (LMP): .... Expected date of delivery (EDD): ....

Educational status:

Husband: .... Wife: ....

Occupation:

Husband: .... Wife: ....

Religion: ....

Labor: 1st stage: .... 2nd stage: .... 3rd stage: ....

ANTENATAL RECORD

Date of Registration: ....

Gestational age at first visit: ....

Sl No.	*Date*	*Weight (kg)*	*Height (cm)*	*Pulse (min)*	*BP (mmHg)*	*Height of Fundus (cm)*	*FHR (mt)*	*Presentation and Position*	*Investigation Done*	*Treatment and Advice Given*

Admission to the Labor Room:

Admission Notes:

- Has been .... hours in labor
- Contraction commenced on .... at ....

- Membranes Intact/Ruptured .... hours ago
- General conditions of the mother: ....

By Palpation:

- Height of the uterus .... weeks
- Condition of the uterus ....
- Position of the fetus ....
- Presentation of the fetus ....
- Abdominal girth ....
- By auscultation ....
- Fetal heart rate (FHR)....................

Vaginal Examination:

- Cervical dilation: ....
- Effacement of the cervix: ....
- Station of the head: ....
- Presentation and position: ....
- Membranes ruptured/intact: ....
- Characteristics of the amniotic fluid: ....
- Pelvis: ....

Delivery Notes:

- Membranes ruptured at: .... AM/PM Spontaneously/Artificially
- Os fully dilated at: .... AM/PM
- Expulsive contraction commenced at: .... AM/PM
- Mode of delivery: ....
- Type of episiotomy: ....
- Baby born at: .... AM/PM on: ....
- Sex of the baby: Male/Female
- Weight of the Baby: .... kg
- Condition of the baby when born: Alive/Asphyxiated/Stillbirth
- Apgar score: ....
- Special observation: Cleft Lip/Cleft Palate/Spina Bifida/Talipes
- Suctioning of the oral and nasal route: ....
- Cord ligation: ....
- Meconium passed: ....
- Initiation of breastfeeding: ....

Partograph

Name Gravida Para Hospital no.

Date of admission Time of admission Ruptured membranes Hours

Fetal heart rate 200 190 180 170 160 150 140 130 120 110 100 90 80

Liquor

moulding

Cervix (cm) (plot X)

Descent of head (plot 0)

10 9 8 7 6 5 4 3 2 1 0

Alert

Action

Hours 1 2 3 4 5 6 7 8 9 10 11 12

Time

Contractions per 10 mins 5 4 3 2 1

Oxytocin U/L

drops/min

Drugs given and IV fluids

Pulse ● and BP ↕ 180 170 160 150 140 130 120 110 100 90 80 70 60

Temp °C

Urine: Protein, Acetone, Volume

DELIVERY OF PLACENTA AND MEMBRANES

- Normal/Manual: .... Removed at: .... AM/PM
- Examination of the placenta: ....
- Weight of the placenta: ....
- Maternal surface: ....
- Type of cord insertion: ....
- Cord length: ....
- Membranes: ....
- Any anatomical variation found: Yes/No
- Specify: ....
- Condition of the perineum: ....
- Any lacerations of the genital passage: Cervix/Vagina/Perineum
- Perineal tear:

  1st Degree: .... 2nd Degree: .... 3rd Degree: .... (Specify if Any)

Drugs Given (name, dosage)	*Route*	*Frequency*	*Action*	*Side Effects*	*Nurses Responsibility*

CONDITION OF THE MOTHER AFTER DELIVERY

Temperature: .... Fundal height: ....

Pulse: .... Uterus: ....

Respiration: .... Vaginal bleeding: ....

Blood pressure: ....

Condition of the neonate: ....

Immediate Care Given:

Needs Identified	*Nursing Care Given*

Conducted by

Assisted by

Signature of the Supervisor

NORMAL DELIVERY CONDUCTED (19)

Hospital: ....

Name of the Mother: ....

Age: .... IP No: ....

Date of Admission: .... Date and Time of Delivery: ....

Booked/Unbooked: .... Mode of Delivery: ....

Date of Booking: .... Date of Discharge: ....

Address: ....

Obstetrical score: ....

Last menstrual period (LMP): .... Expected date of delivery (EDD): ....

Educational status:

Husband: .... Wife: ....

Occupation:

Husband: .... Wife: ....

Religion: ....

Labor: 1st stage: .... 2nd stage: .... 3rd stage: ....

ANTENATAL RECORD

Date of Registration: ....

Gestational age at first visit: ....

Sl No.	*Date*	*Weight (kg)*	*Height (cm)*	*Pulse (min)*	*BP (mmHg)*	*Height of Fundus (cm)*	*FHR (mt)*	*Presentation and Position*	*Investigation Done*	*Treatment and Advice Given*

Admission to the Labor Room:

Admission Notes:

- Has been .... hours in labor
- Contraction commenced on .... at ....

- Membranes Intact/Ruptured .... hours ago
- General conditions of the mother: ....

By Palpation:

- Height of the uterus .... weeks
- Condition of the uterus ....
- Position of the fetus ....
- Presentation of the fetus ....
- Abdominal girth ....
- By auscultation ....
- Fetal heart rate (FHR)..

Vaginal Examination:

- Cervical dilation: ....
- Effacement of the cervix: ....
- Station of the head: ....
- Presentation and position: ....
- Membranes ruptured/intact: ....
- Characteristics of the amniotic fluid: ....
- Pelvis: ....

Delivery Notes:

- Membranes ruptured at: .... AM/PM Spontaneously/Artificially
- Os fully dilated at: .... AM/PM
- Expulsive contraction commenced at: .... AM/PM
- Mode of delivery: ....
- Type of episiotomy: ....
- Baby born at: .... AM/PM on: ....
- Sex of the baby: Male/Female
- Weight of the Baby: .... kg
- Condition of the baby when born: Alive/Asphyxiated/Stillbirth
- Apgar score: ....
- Special observation: Cleft Lip/Cleft Palate/Spina Bifida/Talipes
- Suctioning of the oral and nasal route: ....
- Cord ligation: ....
- Meconium passed: ....
- Initiation of breastfeeding: ....

Partograph

Name Gravida Para Hospital no.

Date of admission Time of admission Ruptured membranes Hours

Fetal heart rate 200 190 180 170 160 150 140 130 120 110 100 90 80

Liquor

moulding

Cervix (cm) (plot X) 10 9 8 7 6 5 4 3 2 1

Descent of head (plot 0)

Alert

Action

Hours 1 2 3 4 5 6 7 8 9 10 11 12

Time 0

Contractions per 10 mins 5 4 3 2 1

Oxytocin U/L

drops/min

Drugs given and IV fluids

Pulse ● and BP ↕ 180 170 160 150 140 130 120 110 100 90 80 70 60

Temp °C

Urine: Protein, Acetone, Volume

DELIVERY OF PLACENTA AND MEMBRANES

- Normal/Manual: .... Removed at: .... AM/PM
- Examination of the placenta: ....
- Weight of the placenta: ....
- Maternal surface: ....
- Type of cord insertion: ....
- Cord length: ....
- Membranes: ....
- Any anatomical variation found: Yes/No
- Specify: ....
- Condition of the perineum: ....
- Any lacerations of the genital passage: Cervix/Vagina/Perineum
- Perineal tear:

  1st Degree: .... 2nd Degree: .... 3rd Degree: .... (Specify if Any)

Drugs Given (name, dosage)	*Route*	*Frequency*	*Action*	*Side Effects*	*Nurses Responsibility*

CONDITION OF THE MOTHER AFTER DELIVERY

Temperature: ....

Fundal height: ....

Pulse: ....

Uterus: ....

Respiration: ....

Vaginal bleeding: ....

Blood pressure: ....

Condition of the neonate: ....

Immediate Care Given:

Needs Identified	*Nursing Care Given*

Conducted by

Assisted by

Signature of the Supervisor

NORMAL DELIVERY CONDUCTED (20)

Hospital: ....

Name of the Mother: ....

Age: .... IP No: ....

Date of Admission: .... Date and Time of Delivery: ....

Booked/Unbooked: .... Mode of Delivery: ....

Date of Booking: .... Date of Discharge: ....

Address: ....

Obstetrical score: ....

Last menstrual period (LMP): .... Expected date of delivery (EDD): ....

Educational status:

Husband: .... Wife: ....

Occupation:

Husband: .... Wife: ....

Religion: ....

Labor: 1st stage: .... 2nd stage: .... 3rd stage: ....

ANTENATAL RECORD

Date of Registration: ....

Gestational age at first visit: ....

Sl No.	*Date*	*Weight (kg)*	*Height (cm)*	*Pulse (min)*	*BP (mmHg)*	*Height of Fundus (cm)*	*FHR (mt)*	*Presentation and Position*	*Investigation Done*	*Treatment and Advice Given*

Admission to the Labor Room:

Admission Notes:

- Has been .... hours in labor
- Contraction commenced on .... at ....

- Membranes Intact/Ruptured .... hours ago
- General conditions of the mother: ....

By Palpation:

- Height of the uterus .... weeks
- Condition of the uterus ....
- Position of the fetus ....
- Presentation of the fetus ....
- Abdominal girth ....
- By auscultation ....
- Fetal heart rate (FHR)..

Vaginal Examination:

- Cervical dilation: ....
- Effacement of the cervix: ....
- Station of the head: ....
- Presentation and position: ....
- Membranes ruptured/intact: ....
- Characteristics of the amniotic fluid: ....
- Pelvis: ....

Delivery Notes:

- Membranes ruptured at: ....AM/PM Spontaneously/Artificially
- Os fully dilated at: .... AM/PM
- Expulsive contraction commenced at: .... AM/PM
- Mode of delivery: ....
- Type of episiotomy: ....
- Baby born at: .... AM/PM on: ....
- Sex of the baby: Male/Female
- Weight of the Baby: .... kg
- Condition of the baby when born: Alive/Asphyxiated/Stillbirth
- Apgar score: ....
- Special observation: Cleft Lip/Cleft Palate/Spina Bifida/Talipes
- Suctioning of the oral and nasal route: ....
- Cord ligation: ....
- Meconium passed: ....
- Initiation of breastfeeding: ....

Partograph

Name Gravida Para Hospital no.

Date of admission Time of admission Ruptured membranes Hours

Fetal heart rate
200 190 180 170 160 150 140 130 120 110 100 90 80

Liquor
moulding

Cervix (cm) (plot X)
Descent of head (plot 0)
10 9 8 7 6 5 4 3 2 1 0

Alert
Action

Hours	1	2	3	4	5	6	7	8	9	10	11	12
Time												

Contractions per 10 mins
5 4 3 2 1

Oxytocin U/L
drops/min

Drugs given and IV fluids

Pulse ●
and
BP ↕
180 170 160 150 140 130 120 110 100 90 80 70 60

Temp °C

Urine
Protein
Acetone
Volume

DELIVERY OF PLACENTA AND MEMBRANES

- Normal/Manual: .... Removed at: .... AM/PM
- Examination of the placenta: ....
- Weight of the placenta: ....
- Maternal surface: ....
- Type of cord insertion: ....
- Cord length: ....
- Membranes: ....
- Any anatomical variation found: Yes/No
- Specify: ....
- Condition of the perineum: ....
- Any lacerations of the genital passage: Cervix/Vagina/Perineum
- Perineal tear:

  1st Degree: .... 2nd Degree: .... 3rd Degree: .... (Specify if Any)

Drugs Given (name, dosage)	*Route*	*Frequency*	*Action*	*Side Effects*	*Nurses Responsibility*

CONDITION OF THE MOTHER AFTER DELIVERY

Temperature: ....

Pulse: ....

Respiration: ....

Blood pressure: ....

Condition of the neonate: ....

Fundal height: ....

Uterus: ....

Vaginal bleeding: ....

Immediate Care Given:

Needs Identified	*Nursing Care Given*

Conducted by

Assisted by

Signature of the Supervisor

CHAPTER 4

Per Vaginal Examination Performed

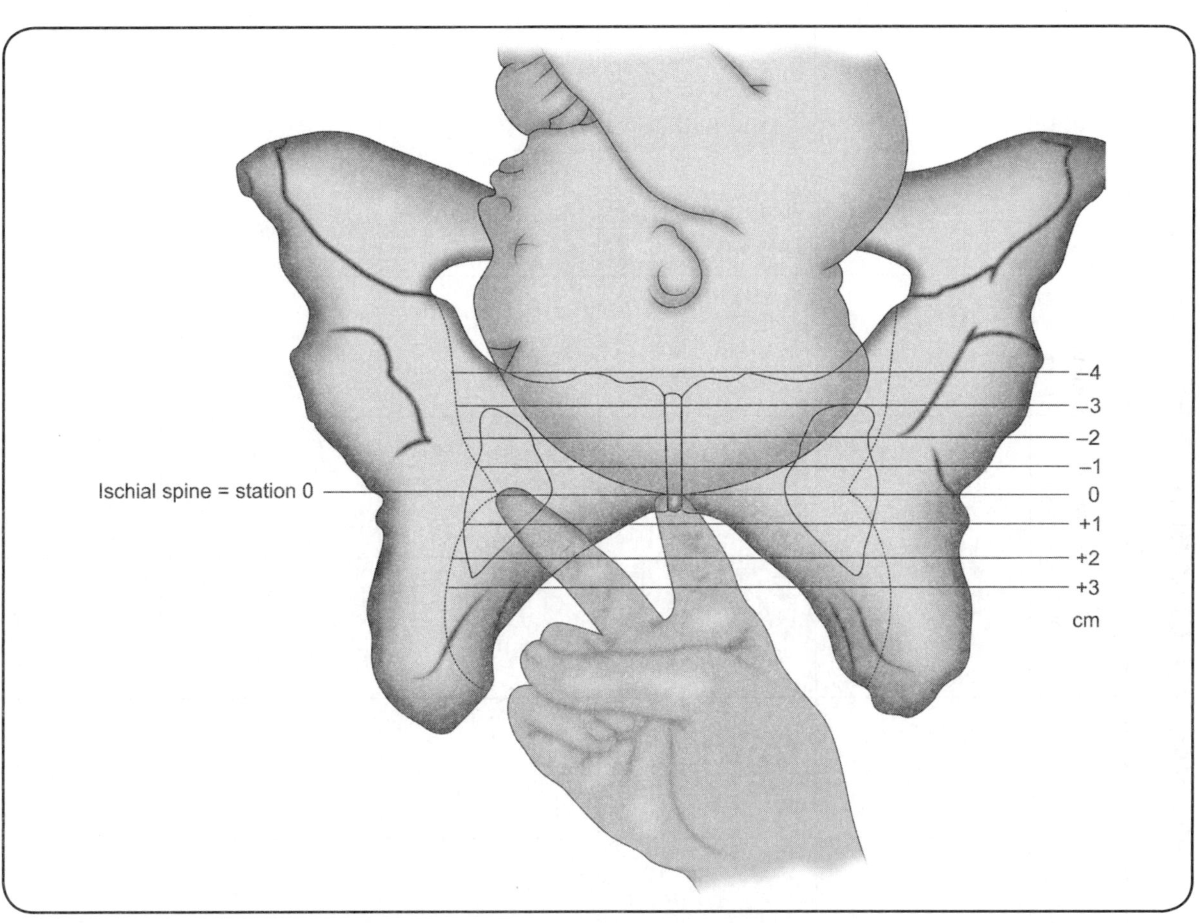

PER VAGINAL EXAMINATION PERFORMED

Sl No.	*IP* No.*	*Name of the Mother*	*GPLSAD*	*LMP*	*EDD*	*Weeks of Gestation*	*Indication for Vaginal Examination*	*Findings*	*Signature of the Students*	*Signature of the Supervisor*
1.										
2.										
3.										
4.										
5.										

*IP, inpatient

CHAPTER 5

Episiotomy Suturing Performed

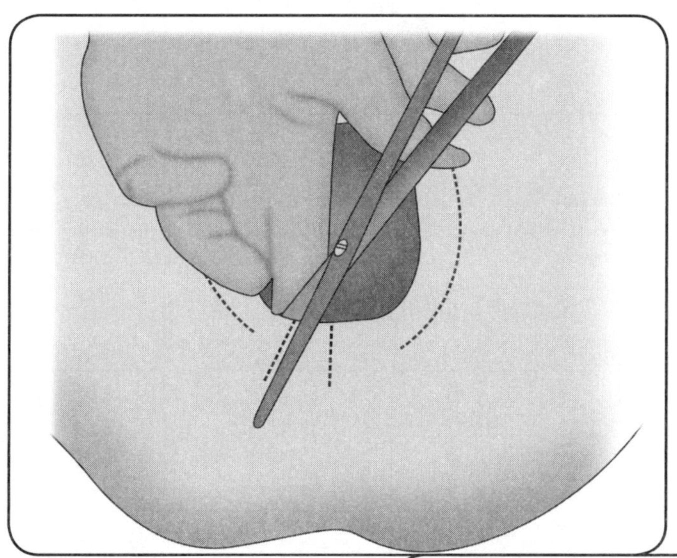

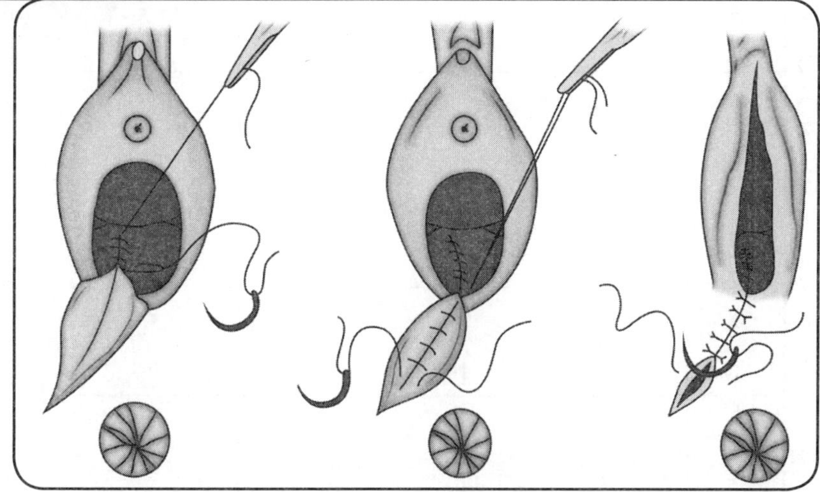

EPISIOTOMY AND SUTURING

Sl No.	*IP* No.*	*Name of the Mother*	*GPLSAD*	*LMP*	*EDD*	*Nature of Delivery*	*Indication for Vaginal Episiotomy*	*Type of Episiotomy Done*	*Condition of the Episiotomy*	*Complications*	*Procedure Done by*	*Supervised by*
1.												
2.												
3.												
4.												
5.												

CHAPTER 6

Postnatal Examination and Care

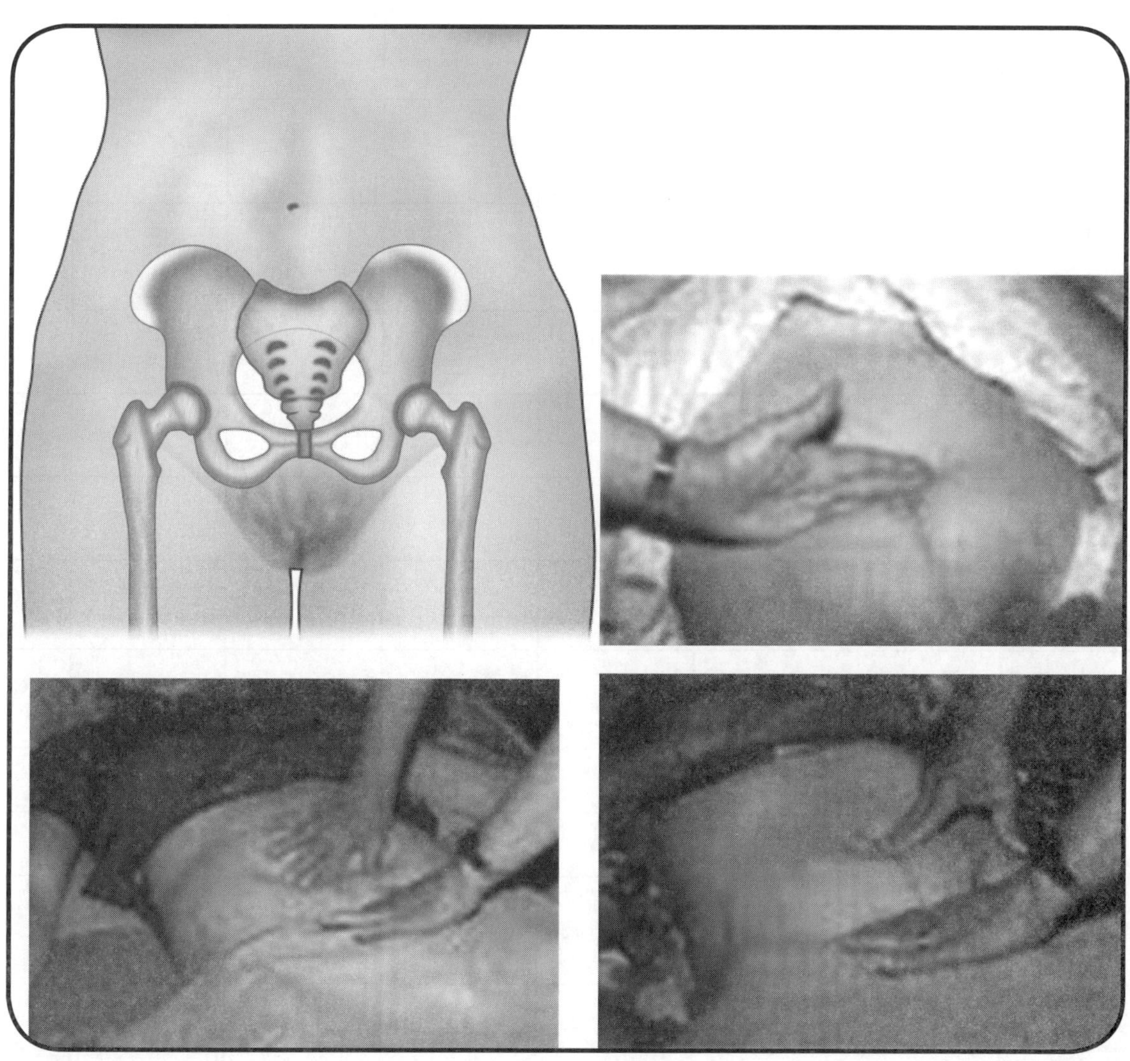

POSTNATAL EXAMINATION AND CARE INCLUDING NEWBORN

Sl No.	*IP No.*	*Name of the Mother*	*Age*	*Obstetrical Score*	*LMP*	*EDD*	*Type of Delivery*	*Condition of the Mother*					*Condition of the Baby*			*Treatment and Advice Given*
								BP (mm Hg)	*Pulse (min)*	*Fundal Height (cm)*	*Lochia*	*Episiotomy*	*Suturing*	*Weight Sex*	*Apgar Score*	
1.																
2.																
3.																
4.																
5.																
6.																
7.																

8.																
9.																
10.																
11.																
12.																
13.																
14.																
15.																

POSTNATAL EXAMINATION AND CARE (1)

Profile	*Mother*	*Father*
Name		
Age		
Educational status		
Occupation		
Religion		
Address		

OP/IP No.												
Date of admission												
EDD												
LMP												
Obstetrical score	G		P		L		A		S		D	
Weeks of gestation												
Date and time of delivery												
Type of delivery												
Sex of baby												
Weight of baby												
Postnatal day												
Date of discharge												

1. Socioeconomic Status:
   a. Total income of the family: ....
   b. Living standard:
   c. Type of the house:
      - Ownership of the House: ....
        Own/Rented: ....
        Number of rooms: ....
      - Environmental condition of the house:
        Lighting facility: ....
        Water facility: ....
        Drainage: ....
        Kitchen garden: ....
        Pet animals: ....

2. Family History:

Type of family: Nuclear Family/Joint Family

Sl No.	*Name of the Family Members*	*Age*	*Sex*	*Educational Status*	*Occupational Status*	*Relationship with the Mother*	*Health Status*
1.							
2.							
3.							
4.							
5.							
6.							
7.							
8.							
9.							

History of Any:

a. Communicable disease: ....

b. Hereditary diseases: ....

c. Twin pregnancy/Bad obstetrical history: ....

3. Personal History:

a. Dietary pattern: ....

b. Sleeping pattern: ....

c. Habits: ....

d. Bowel elimination: ....

e. Bladder elimination: ....

f. Immunization history: ....

g. Sexual history: ....

h. Drugs history: .... Drug allergy: ....

4. Menstrual History: ....

5. Marital History: ....

6. Contraceptive History: ....

7. Previous Medical and Surgical History: ....

8. Previous Obstetrical History: ....

Sl No.	*Year*	*Antenatal Period*	*Intranatal Period*	*Postnatal Period*	*Baby*			*Remarks*
					Alive/Stillbirth	*Sex*	*Weight (kg)*	

9. Present Obstetrical History: ....

Antenatal period: ....

Intranatal period: ....

Postnatal period: ....

a. Physical Examination:

- General condition:
- General appearance:

  Body built: .... Health status: ....

  Activity: ....

  Head: .... Hair: ....

- Facial appearance:

  Eyes: .... Ears: ....

  Nose: ....

- Mouth:

  Gums: .... Teeth: ....

  Tongue: .... Tonsils: ....

- Neck: ....

- Upper limbs:
- Chest: .... Lungs: ....

  Heart: ....
- Vital signs:

  Temperature: .... Pulse: ....

  Respiration: .... Blood pressure: ....

b. Obstetrical Examination:

- Breast:

  Size: .... Primary areola: ....

  Montgomery's tubercles: .... Secondary areola: ....

  Colostrums: .... Consistency: ....

  Discolorations: .... Any other: ....
- Uterus:

  Palpation: .... Fundal height: ....
- Bladder:

  Nipple protractility: .... Nodules/Lumps: ....
- Normal/Incontinence/Retention/Residual: ....
- Bowel sound: ....

  Bowel movement: ....

  Normal/Constipation/Loose Stool: ....
- Perineum:

  Condition: ....

  Intact/Laceration/Degree of Tear/Episiotomy: ....

  Assessment of Episiotomy/Tear: ....

  Lochia: .... Color: ....

  Rubra/Serosa/Alba Amount: ....

  Odor: ....
- Extremities:

  Range of joint movement: .... Pain: ....

  Discoloration: .... Any other: ....

ASSESSMENT OF THE NEWBORN

Name of the Baby: ....

Age of the Baby: .... Weight of the Baby: ....

Apgar Score: 1 Minute: .... 5 Minutes: ....

1. Anthropometric Measurement:

   Length: .... Weight: ....

   Head circumference: .... Chest circumference: ....

2. Vital Signs:

   Temperature: .... Heart rate: ....

   Respiration: ....

3. General Assessment:

   Activity: ....

   Head: ....

   Eyes: ....

   Ears: ....

   Mouth: ....

   Nose: ....

   Neck: ....

   Chest: ....

   Abdomen: ....

   Spine: ....

   Anus: ....

   Extremities: ....

4. Reflexes:

   Moro reflexes: ....

   Tonic neck reflexes: ....

   Feeding Reflexes: ....

   Rooting reflexes: .... Sucking reflexes: ....

   Swallowing reflexes: .... Gag reflexes: ....

   Blinking: ....

   Yawn: ....

   Protective Reflexes: ....

5. Elimination:

   Urine output: .... Cough and sneeze: ....

   Meconium: ....

NURSING CARE PLAN

Assessment	*Nursing Diagnosis*	*Goals*	*Nursing Intervention*	*Rationale*	*Nursing Implementation*	*Evaluation*

NURSING CARE PLAN

Assessment	*Nursing Diagnosis*	*Goals*	*Nursing Intervention*	*Rationale*	*Nursing Implementation*	*Evaluation*

NURSING CARE PLAN

Assessment	*Nursing Diagnosis*	*Goals*	*Nursing Intervention*	*Rationale*	*Nursing Implementation*	*Evaluation*

CLINICAL CHART OF PUERPERIUM

Date											
Temperature (°F)											*Fundal Height (cm)*
106											20
105											18
104											16
103											14
101											12
100											10
99											8
98											6
95											4
94											2
93											1
Pulse/mt											
BP (mm Hg)											
Respiration/mt											
Urine Output											
Bowel Examination											
Lochia											
Perineal Care											
Episiotomy Wound Healing											
Breastfeeding (Conditions of the Breast)											
Chief Complaints											
Treatment Given											

POSTNATAL EXAMINATION AND CARE (2)

Profile	*Mother*	*Father*
Name		
Age		
Educational status		
Occupation		
Religion		
Address		

OP/IP No.												
Date of admission												
EDD												
LMP												
Obstetrical score	G		P		L		A		S		D	
Weeks of gestation												
Date and time of delivery												
Type of delivery												
Sex of baby												
Weight of baby												
Postnatal day												
Date of discharge												

1. Socioeconomic Status:
   a. Total income of the family: ....
   b. Living standard:
   c. Type of the house:
      - Ownership of the House: ....
        Own/Rented: ....
        Number of rooms: ....
      - Environmental condition of the house:
        Lighting facility: ....
        Water facility: ....
        Drainage: ....
        Kitchen garden: ....
        Pet animals: ....

2. Family History:

   Type of family: Nuclear Family/Joint Family

Sl No.	*Name of the Family Members*	*Age*	*Sex*	*Educational Status*	*Occupational Status*	*Relationship with the Mother*	*Health Status*
1.							
2.							
3.							
4.							
5.							
6.							
7.							
8.							
9.							

   History of Any:

   a. Communicable disease: ....

   b. Hereditary diseases: ....

   c. Twin pregnancy/Bad obstetrical history: ....

3. Personal History:

   a. Dietary pattern: ....

   b. Sleeping pattern: ....

   c. Habits: ....

   d. Bowel elimination: ....

   e. Bladder elimination: ....

   f. Immunization history: ....

   g. Sexual history: ....

   h. Drugs history: .... Drug allergy: ....

4. Menstrual History: ....

5. Marital History: ....

6. Contraceptive History: ....

7. Previous Medical and Surgical History: ....

8. Previous Obstetrical History: ....

Sl No.	Year	Antenatal Period	Intranatal Period	Postnatal Period	Baby			Remarks
					Alive/Stillbirth	Sex	Weight (kg)	

9. Present Obstetrical History: ....

Antenatal period: ....

Intranatal period: ....

Postnatal period: ....

a. Physical Examination:

- General condition:
- General appearance:

  Body built: .... Health status: ....

  Activity: ....

  Head: .... Hair: ....

- Facial appearance:

  Eyes: .... Ears: ....

  Nose: ....

- Mouth:

  Gums: .... Teeth: ....

  Tongue: .... Tonsils: ....

- Neck: ....

- Upper limbs:
- Chest: .... Lungs: ....

  Heart: ....
- Vital signs:

  Temperature: .... Pulse: ....

  Respiration: .... Blood pressure: ....

b. Obstetrical Examination:

- Breast:

  Size: .... Primary areola: ....

  Montgomery's tubercles: .... Secondary areola: ....

  Colostrums: .... Consistency: ....

  Discolorations: .... Any other: ....
- Uterus:

  Palpation: .... Fundal height: ....
- Bladder:

  Nipple protractility: .... Nodules/Lumps: ....
- Normal/Incontinence/Retention/Residual: ....
- Bowel sound: ....

  Bowel movement: ....

  Normal/Constipation/Loose Stool: ....
- Perineum:

  Condition: ....

  Intact/Laceration/Degree of Tear/Episiotomy: ....

  Assessment of Episiotomy/Tear: ....

  Lochia: .... Color: ....

  Rubra/Serosa/Alba Amount: ....

  Odor: ....
- Extremities:

  Range of joint movement: .... Pain: ....

  Discoloration: .... Any other: ....

ASSESSMENT OF THE NEWBORN

Name of the Baby: ....

Age of the Baby: .... Weight of the Baby: ....

Apgar Score: 1 Minute: .... 5 Minutes: ....

1. Anthropometric Measurement:

   Length: .... Weight: ....

   Head circumference: .... Chest circumference: ....

2. Vital Signs:

   Temperature: .... Heart rate: ....

   Respiration: ....

3. General Assessment:

   Activity: ....

   Head: ....

   Eyes: ....

   Ears: ....

   Mouth: ....

   Nose: ....

   Neck: ....

   Chest: ....

   Abdomen: ....

   Spine: ....

   Anus: ....

   Extremities: ....

4. Reflexes:

   Moro reflexes: ....

   Tonic neck reflexes: ....

   Feeding Reflexes: ....

   Rooting reflexes: .... Sucking reflexes: ....

   Swallowing reflexes: .... Gag reflexes: ....

   Blinking: ....

   Yawn: ....

   Protective Reflexes: ....

5. Elimination:

   Urine output: .... Cough and sneeze: ....

   Meconium: ....

NURSING CARE PLAN

Assessment	*Nursing Diagnosis*	*Goals*	*Nursing Intervention*	*Rationale*	*Nursing Implementation*	*Evaluation*

NURSING CARE PLAN

Assessment	*Nursing Diagnosis*	*Goals*	*Nursing Intervention*	*Rationale*	*Nursing Implementation*	*Evaluation*

NURSING CARE PLAN

Assessment	*Nursing Diagnosis*	*Goals*	*Nursing Intervention*	*Rationale*	*Nursing Implementation*	*Evaluation*

CLINICAL CHART OF PUERPERIUM

Date											
Temperature (°F)											*Fundal Height (cm)*
106											20
105											18
104											16
103											14
101											12
100											10
99											8
98											6
95											4
94											2
93											1
Pulse/mt											
BP (mm Hg)											
Respiration/mt											
Urine Output											
Bowel Examination											
Lochia											
Perineal Care											
Episiotomy Wound Healing											
Breastfeeding (Conditions of the Breast)											
Chief Complaints											
Treatment Given											

POSTNATAL EXAMINATION AND CARE (3)

Profile	*Mother*	*Father*
Name		
Age		
Educational status		
Occupation		
Religion		
Address		

OP/IP No.												
Date of admission												
EDD												
LMP												
Obstetrical score	G		P		L		A		S		D	
Weeks of gestation												
Date and time of delivery												
Type of delivery												
Sex of baby												
Weight of baby												
Postnatal day												
Date of discharge												

1. Socioeconomic Status:
   a. Total income of the family: ....
   b. Living standard:
   c. Type of the house:
      - Ownership of the House: ....
        Own/Rented: ....
        Number of rooms: ....
      - Environmental condition of the house:
        Lighting facility: ....
        Water facility: ....
        Drainage: ....
        Kitchen garden: ....
        Pet animals: ....

2. Family History:

   Type of family: Nuclear Family/Joint Family

Sl No.	*Name of the Family Members*	*Age*	*Sex*	*Educational Status*	*Occupational Status*	*Relationship with the Mother*	*Health Status*
1.							
2.							
3.							
4.							
5.							
6.							
7.							
8.							
9.							

   History of Any:

   a. Communicable disease: ....

   b. Hereditary diseases: ....

   c. Twin pregnancy/Bad obstetrical history: ....

3. Personal History:

   a. Dietary pattern: ....

   b. Sleeping pattern: ....

   c. Habits: ....

   d. Bowel elimination: ....

   e. Bladder elimination: ....

   f. Immunization history: ....

   g. Sexual history: ....

   h. Drugs history: .... Drug allergy: ....

4. Menstrual History: ....

5. Marital History: ....

6. Contraceptive History: ....

7. Previous Medical and Surgical History: ....

8. Previous Obstetrical History: ....

Sl No.	Year	Antenatal Period	Intranatal Period	Postnatal Period	Baby			Remarks
					Alive/Stillbirth	Sex	Weight (kg)	

9. Present Obstetrical History: ....

Antenatal period: ....

Intranatal period: ....

Postnatal period: ....

a. Physical Examination:
   - General condition:
   - General appearance:

     Body built: .... Health status: ....

     Activity: ....

     Head: .... Hair: ....
   - Facial appearance:

     Eyes: .... Ears: ....

     Nose: ....
   - Mouth:

     Gums: .... Teeth: ....

     Tongue: .... Tonsils: ....
   - Neck: ....

- Upper limbs:
- Chest: .... Lungs: ....

  Heart: ....
- Vital signs:

  Temperature: .... Pulse: ....

  Respiration: .... Blood pressure: ....

b. Obstetrical Examination:

- Breast:

  Size: .... Primary areola: ....

  Montgomery's tubercles: .... Secondary areola: ....

  Colostrums: .... Consistency: ....

  Discolorations: .... Any other: ....
- Uterus:

  Palpation: .... Fundal height: ....
- Bladder:

  Nipple protractility: .... Nodules/Lumps: ....
- Normal/Incontinence/Retention/Residual: ....
- Bowel sound: ....

  Bowel movement: ....

  Normal/Constipation/Loose Stool: ....
- Perineum:

  Condition: ....

  Intact/Laceration/Degree of Tear/Episiotomy: ....

  Assessment of Episiotomy/Tear: ....

  Lochia: .... Color: ....

  Rubra/Serosa/Alba Amount: ....

  Odor: ....
- Extremities:

  Range of joint movement: .... Pain: ....

  Discoloration: .... Any other: ....

ASSESSMENT OF THE NEWBORN

Name of the Baby: ....

Age of the Baby: .... Weight of the Baby: ....

Apgar Score: 1 Minute: .... 5 Minutes: ....

1. Anthropometric Measurement:

   Length: .... Weight: ....

   Head circumference: .... Chest circumference: ....

2. Vital Signs:

   Temperature: .... Heart rate: ....

   Respiration: ....

3. General Assessment:

   Activity: ....

   Head: ....

   Eyes: ....

   Ears: ....

   Mouth: ....

   Nose: ....

   Neck: ....

   Chest: ....

   Abdomen: ....

   Spine: ....

   Anus: ....

   Extremities: ....

4. Reflexes:

   Moro reflexes: ....

   Tonic neck reflexes: ....

   Feeding Reflexes: ....

   Rooting reflexes: .... Sucking reflexes: ....

   Swallowing reflexes: .... Gag reflexes: ....

   Blinking: ....

   Yawn: ....

   Protective Reflexes: ....

5. Elimination:

   Urine output: .... Cough and sneeze: ....

   Meconium: ....

NURSING CARE PLAN

Assessment	*Nursing Diagnosis*	*Goals*	*Nursing Intervention*	*Rationale*	*Nursing Implementation*	*Evaluation*

NURSING CARE PLAN

Assessment	*Nursing Diagnosis*	*Goals*	*Nursing Intervention*	*Rationale*	*Nursing Implementation*	*Evaluation*

NURSING CARE PLAN

Assessment	Nursing Diagnosis	Goals	Nursing Intervention	Rationale	Nursing Implementation	Evaluation

CLINICAL CHART OF PUERPERIUM

Date											
Temperature (°F)											*Fundal Height (cm)*
106											20
105											18
104											16
103											14
101											12
100											10
99											8
98											6
95											4
94											2
93											1
Pulse/mt											
BP (mm Hg)											
Respiration/mt											
Urine Output											
Bowel Examination											
Lochia											
Perineal Care											
Episiotomy Wound Healing											
Breastfeeding (Conditions of the Breast)											
Chief Complaints											
Treatment Given											

POSTNATAL EXAMINATION AND CARE (4)

Profile	*Mother*	*Father*
Name		
Age		
Educational status		
Occupation		
Religion		
Address		

OP/IP No.												
Date of admission												
EDD												
LMP												
Obstetrical score	G		P		L		A		S		D	
Weeks of gestation												
Date and time of delivery												
Type of delivery												
Sex of baby												
Weight of baby												
Postnatal day												
Date of discharge												

1. Socioeconomic Status:
   a. Total income of the family: ....
   b. Living standard:
   c. Type of the house:
      - Ownership of the House: ....
        Own/Rented: ....
        Number of rooms: ....
      - Environmental condition of the house:
        Lighting facility: ....
        Water facility: ....
        Drainage: ....
        Kitchen garden: ....
        Pet animals: ....

2. Family History:

   Type of family: Nuclear Family/Joint Family

Sl No.	*Name of the Family Members*	*Age*	*Sex*	*Educational Status*	*Occupational Status*	*Relationship with the Mother*	*Health Status*
1.							
2.							
3.							
4.							
5.							
6.							
7.							
8.							
9.							

   History of Any:

   a. Communicable disease: ....

   b. Hereditary diseases: ....

   c. Twin pregnancy/Bad obstetrical history: ....

3. Personal History:

   a. Dietary pattern: ....

   b. Sleeping pattern: ....

   c. Habits: ....

   d. Bowel elimination: ....

   e. Bladder elimination: ....

   f. Immunization history: ....

   g. Sexual history: ....

   h. Drugs history: .... Drug allergy: ....

4. Menstrual History: ....

5. Marital History: ....

6. Contraceptive History: ....

7. Previous Medical and Surgical History: ....

8. Previous Obstetrical History: ....

Sl No.	*Year*	*Antenatal Period*	*Intranatal Period*	*Postnatal Period*	*Baby*			*Remarks*
					Alive/Stillbirth	*Sex*	*Weight (kg)*	

9. Present Obstetrical History: ....

Antenatal period: ....

Intranatal period: ....

Postnatal period: ....

a. Physical Examination:

- General condition:
- General appearance:

  Body built: .... Health status: ....

  Activity: ....

  Head: .... Hair: ....
- Facial appearance:

  Eyes: .... Ears: ....

  Nose: ....
- Mouth:

  Gums: .... Teeth: ....

  Tongue: .... Tonsils: ....
- Neck: ....

- Upper limbs:
- Chest: .... Lungs: ....

  Heart: ....
- Vital signs:

  Temperature: .... Pulse: ....

  Respiration: .... Blood pressure: ....

b. Obstetrical Examination:

- Breast:

  Size: .... Primary areola: ....

  Montgomery's tubercles: .... Secondary areola: ....

  Colostrums: .... Consistency: ....

  Discolorations: .... Any other: ....
- Uterus:

  Palpation: .... Fundal height: ....
- Bladder:

  Nipple protractility: .... Nodules/Lumps: ....
- Normal/Incontinence/Retention/Residual: ....
- Bowel sound: ....

  Bowel movement: ....

  Normal/Constipation/Loose Stool: ....
- Perineum:

  Condition: ....

  Intact/Laceration/Degree of Tear/Episiotomy: ....

  Assessment of Episiotomy/Tear: ....

  Lochia: .... Color: ....

  Rubra/Serosa/Alba Amount: ....

  Odor: ....
- Extremities:

  Range of joint movement: .... Pain: ....

  Discoloration: .... Any other: ....

ASSESSMENT OF THE NEWBORN

Name of the Baby: ....

Age of the Baby: .... Weight of the Baby: ....

Apgar Score: 1 Minute: .... 5 Minutes: ....

1. Anthropometric Measurement:

   Length: .... Weight: ....

   Head circumference: .... Chest circumference: ....

2. Vital Signs:

   Temperature: .... Heart rate: ....

   Respiration: ....

3. General Assessment:

   Activity: ....

   Head: ....

   Eyes: ....

   Ears: ....

   Mouth: ....

   Nose: ....

   Neck: ....

   Chest: ....

   Abdomen: ....

   Spine: ....

   Anus: ....

   Extremities: ....

4. Reflexes:

   Moro reflexes: ....

   Tonic neck reflexes: ....

   Feeding Reflexes: ....

   Rooting reflexes: .... Sucking reflexes: ....

   Swallowing reflexes: .... Gag reflexes: ....

   Blinking: ....

   Yawn: ....

   Protective Reflexes: ....

5. Elimination:

   Urine output: .... Cough and sneeze: ....

   Meconium: ....

NURSING CARE PLAN

Assessment	*Nursing Diagnosis*	*Goals*	*Nursing Intervention*	*Rationale*	*Nursing Implementation*	*Evaluation*

NURSING CARE PLAN

Assessment	*Nursing Diagnosis*	*Goals*	*Nursing Intervention*	*Rationale*	*Nursing Implementation*	*Evaluation*

NURSING CARE PLAN

Assessment	*Nursing Diagnosis*	*Goals*	*Nursing Intervention*	*Rationale*	*Nursing Implementation*	*Evaluation*

CLINICAL CHART OF PUERPERIUM

Date											
Temperature (°F)											*Fundal Height (cm)*
106											20
105											18
104											16
103											14
101											12
100											10
99											8
98											6
95											4
94											2
93											1
Pulse/mt											
BP (mm Hg)											
Respiration/mt											
Urine Output											
Bowel Examination											
Lochia											
Perineal Care											
Episiotomy Wound Healing											
Breastfeeding (Conditions of the Breast)											
Chief Complaints											
Treatment Given											

POSTNATAL EXAMINATION AND CARE (5)

Profile	*Mother*	*Father*
Name		
Age		
Educational status		
Occupation		
Religion		
Address		

OP/IP No.												
Date of admission												
EDD												
LMP												
Obstetrical score	G		P		L		A		S		D	
Weeks of gestation												
Date and time of delivery												
Type of delivery												
Sex of baby												
Weight of baby												
Postnatal day												
Date of discharge												

1. Socioeconomic Status:
   a. Total income of the family: ....
   b. Living standard:
   c. Type of the house:
      - Ownership of the House: ....
        Own/Rented: ....
        Number of rooms: ....
      - Environmental condition of the house:
        Lighting facility: ....
        Water facility: ....
        Drainage: ....
        Kitchen garden: ....
        Pet animals: ....

2. Family History:

   Type of family: Nuclear Family/Joint Family

Sl No.	*Name of the Family Members*	*Age*	*Sex*	*Educational Status*	*Occupational Status*	*Relationship with the Mother*	*Health Status*
1.							
2.							
3.							
4.							
5.							
6.							
7.							
8.							
9.							

   History of Any:

   a. Communicable disease: ....

   b. Hereditary diseases: ....

   c. Twin pregnancy/Bad obstetrical history: ....

3. Personal History:

   a. Dietary pattern: ....

   b. Sleeping pattern: ....

   c. Habits: ....

   d. Bowel elimination: ....

   e. Bladder elimination: ....

   f. Immunization history: ....

   g. Sexual history: ....

   h. Drugs history: .... Drug allergy: ....

4. Menstrual History: ....

5. Marital History: ....

6. Contraceptive History: ....

7. Previous Medical and Surgical History: ....

8. Previous Obstetrical History: ....

Sl No.	*Year*	*Antenatal Period*	*Intranatal Period*	*Postnatal Period*	*Baby*			*Remarks*
					Alive/Stillbirth	*Sex*	*Weight (kg)*	

9. Present Obstetrical History: ....

Antenatal period: ....

Intranatal period: ....

Postnatal period: ....

a. Physical Examination:

- General condition:
- General appearance:

  Body built: .... Health status: ....

  Activity: ....

  Head: .... Hair: ....
- Facial appearance:

  Eyes: .... Ears: ....

  Nose: ....
- Mouth:

  Gums: .... Teeth: ....

  Tongue: .... Tonsils: ....
- Neck: ....

- Upper limbs:
- Chest: .... Lungs: ....

  Heart: ....
- Vital signs:

  Temperature: .... Pulse: ....

  Respiration: .... Blood pressure: ....

b. Obstetrical Examination:

- Breast:

  Size: .... Primary areola: ....

  Montgomery's tubercles: .... Secondary areola: ....

  Colostrums: .... Consistency: ....

  Discolorations: .... Any other: ....
- Uterus:

  Palpation: .... Fundal height: ....
- Bladder:

  Nipple protractility: .... Nodules/Lumps: ....
- Normal/Incontinence/Retention/Residual: ....
- Bowel sound: ....

  Bowel movement: ....

  Normal/Constipation/Loose Stool: ....
- Perineum:

  Condition: ....

  Intact/Laceration/Degree of Tear/Episiotomy: ....

  Assessment of Episiotomy/Tear: ....

  Lochia: .... Color: ....

  Rubra/Serosa/Alba Amount: ....

  Odor: ....
- Extremities:

  Range of joint movement: .... Pain: ....

  Discoloration: .... Any other: ....

ASSESSMENT OF THE NEWBORN

Name of the Baby: ....

Age of the Baby: .... Weight of the Baby: ....

Apgar Score: 1 Minute: .... 5 Minutes: ....

1. Anthropometric Measurement:
   Length: .... Weight: ....
   Head circumference: .... Chest circumference: ....
2. Vital Signs:
   Temperature: .... Heart rate: ....
   Respiration: ....
3. General Assessment:
   Activity: ....
   Head: ....
   Eyes: ....
   Ears: ....
   Mouth: ....
   Nose: ....
   Neck: ....
   Chest: ....
   Abdomen: ....
   Spine: ....
   Anus: ....
   Extremities: ....
4. Reflexes:
   Moro reflexes: ....
   Tonic neck reflexes: ....
   Feeding Reflexes: ....
   Rooting reflexes: .... Sucking reflexes: ....
   Swallowing reflexes: .... Gag reflexes: ....
   Blinking: ....
   Yawn: ....
   Protective Reflexes: ....
5. Elimination:
   Urine output: .... Cough and sneeze: ....
   Meconium: ....

NURSING CARE PLAN

Assessment	*Nursing Diagnosis*	*Goals*	*Nursing Intervention*	*Rationale*	*Nursing Implementation*	*Evaluation*

NURSING CARE PLAN

Assessment	Nursing Diagnosis	Goals	Nursing Intervention	Rationale	Nursing Implementation	Evaluation

NURSING CARE PLAN

Assessment	*Nursing Diagnosis*	*Goals*	*Nursing Intervention*	*Rationale*	*Nursing Implementation*	*Evaluation*

CLINICAL CHART OF PUERPERIUM

Date											
Temperature (°F)											*Fundal Height (cm)*
106											20
105											18
104											16
103											14
101											12
100											10
99											8
98											6
95											4
94											2
93											1
Pulse/mt											
BP (mm Hg)											
Respiration/mt											
Urine Output											
Bowel Examination											
Lochia											
Perineal Care											
Episiotomy Wound Healing											
Breastfeeding (Conditions of the Breast)											
Chief Complaints											
Treatment Given											

POSTNATAL EXAMINATION AND CARE (6)

Profile	*Mother*	*Father*
Name		
Age		
Educational status		
Occupation		
Religion		
Address		

OP/IP No.												
Date of admission												
EDD												
LMP												
Obstetrical score	G		P		L		A		S		D	
Weeks of gestation												
Date and time of delivery												
Type of delivery												
Sex of baby												
Weight of baby												
Postnatal day												
Date of discharge												

1. Socioeconomic Status:
   a. Total income of the family: ....
   b. Living standard:
   c. Type of the house:
      - Ownership of the House: ....
        Own/Rented: ....
        Number of rooms: ....
      - Environmental condition of the house:
        Lighting facility: ....
        Water facility: ....
        Drainage: ....
        Kitchen garden: ....
        Pet animals: ....

2. Family History:

   Type of family: Nuclear Family/Joint Family

Sl No.	*Name of the Family Members*	*Age*	*Sex*	*Educational Status*	*Occupational Status*	*Relationship with the Mother*	*Health Status*
1.							
2.							
3.							
4.							
5.							
6.							
7.							
8.							
9.							

   History of Any:

   a. Communicable disease: ....

   b. Hereditary diseases: ....

   c. Twin pregnancy/Bad obstetrical history: ....

3. Personal History:

   a. Dietary pattern: ....

   b. Sleeping pattern: ....

   c. Habits: ....

   d. Bowel elimination: ....

   e. Bladder elimination: ....

   f. Immunization history: ....

   g. Sexual history: ....

   h. Drugs history: .... Drug allergy: ....

4. Menstrual History: ....

5. Marital History: ....

6. Contraceptive History: ....

7. Previous Medical and Surgical History: ....

8. Previous Obstetrical History: ....

Sl No.	*Year*	*Antenatal Period*	*Intranatal Period*	*Postnatal Period*	*Baby*			*Remarks*
					Alive/Stillbirth	*Sex*	*Weight (kg)*	

9. Present Obstetrical History: ....

Antenatal period: ....

Intranatal period: ....

Postnatal period: ....

a. Physical Examination:

- General condition:
- General appearance:

  Body built: .... Health status: ....

  Activity: ....

  Head: .... Hair: ....
- Facial appearance:

  Eyes: .... Ears: ....

  Nose: ....
- Mouth:

  Gums: .... Teeth: ....

  Tongue: .... Tonsils: ....
- Neck: ....

- Upper limbs:
- Chest: .... Lungs: ....

  Heart: ....
- Vital signs:

  Temperature: .... Pulse: ....

  Respiration: .... Blood pressure: ....

b. Obstetrical Examination:

- Breast:

  Size: .... Primary areola: ....

  Montgomery's tubercles: .... Secondary areola: ....

  Colostrums: .... Consistency: ....

  Discolorations: .... Any other: ....
- Uterus:

  Palpation: .... Fundal height: ....
- Bladder:

  Nipple protractility: .... Nodules/Lumps: ....
- Normal/Incontinence/Retention/Residual: ....
- Bowel sound: ....

  Bowel movement: ....

  Normal/Constipation/Loose Stool: ....
- Perineum:

  Condition: ....

  Intact/Laceration/Degree of Tear/Episiotomy: ....

  Assessment of Episiotomy/Tear: ....

  Lochia: .... Color: ....

  Rubra/Serosa/Alba Amount: ....

  Odor: ....
- Extremities:

  Range of joint movement: .... Pain: ....

  Discoloration: .... Any other: ....

ASSESSMENT OF THE NEWBORN

Name of the Baby: ....

Age of the Baby: .... Weight of the Baby: ....

Apgar Score: 1 Minute: .... 5 Minutes: ....

1. Anthropometric Measurement:

   Length: .... Weight: ....

   Head circumference: .... Chest circumference: ....

2. Vital Signs:

   Temperature: .... Heart rate: ....

   Respiration: ....

3. General Assessment:

   Activity: ....

   Head: ....

   Eyes: ....

   Ears: ....

   Mouth: ....

   Nose: ....

   Neck: ....

   Chest: ....

   Abdomen: ....

   Spine: ....

   Anus: ....

   Extremities: ....

4. Reflexes:

   Moro reflexes: ....

   Tonic neck reflexes: ....

   Feeding Reflexes: ....

   Rooting reflexes: .... Sucking reflexes: ....

   Swallowing reflexes: .... Gag reflexes: ....

   Blinking: ....

   Yawn: ....

   Protective Reflexes: ....

5. Elimination:

   Urine output: .... Cough and sneeze: ....

   Meconium: ....

NURSING CARE PLAN

Assessment	*Nursing Diagnosis*	*Goals*	*Nursing Intervention*	*Rationale*	*Nursing Implementation*	*Evaluation*

NURSING CARE PLAN

Assessment	*Nursing Diagnosis*	*Goals*	*Nursing Intervention*	*Rationale*	*Nursing Implementation*	*Evaluation*

NURSING CARE PLAN

Assessment	*Nursing Diagnosis*	*Goals*	*Nursing Intervention*	*Rationale*	*Nursing Implementation*	*Evaluation*

CLINICAL CHART OF PUERPERIUM

Date											
Temperature (°F)											*Fundal Height (cm)*
106											20
105											18
104											16
103											14
101											12
100											10
99											8
98											6
95											4
94											2
93											1
Pulse/mt											
BP (mm Hg)											
Respiration/mt											
Urine Output											
Bowel Examination											
Lochia											
Perineal Care											
Episiotomy Wound Healing											
Breastfeeding (Conditions of the Breast)											
Chief Complaints											
Treatment Given											

POSTNATAL EXAMINATION AND CARE (7)

Profile	*Mother*	*Father*
Name		
Age		
Educational status		
Occupation		
Religion		
Address		

OP/IP No.												
Date of admission												
EDD												
LMP												
Obstetrical score	G		P		L		A		S		D	
Weeks of gestation												
Date and time of delivery												
Type of delivery												
Sex of baby												
Weight of baby												
Postnatal day												
Date of discharge												

1. Socioeconomic Status:
   a. Total income of the family: ....
   b. Living standard:
   c. Type of the house:
      - Ownership of the House: ....
        Own/Rented: ....
        Number of rooms: ....
      - Environmental condition of the house:
        Lighting facility: ....
        Water facility: ....
        Drainage: ....
        Kitchen garden: ....
        Pet animals: ....

2. Family History:

   Type of family: Nuclear Family/Joint Family

Sl No.	*Name of the Family Members*	*Age*	*Sex*	*Educational Status*	*Occupational Status*	*Relationship with the Mother*	*Health Status*
1.							
2.							
3.							
4.							
5.							
6.							
7.							
8.							
9.							

   History of Any:

   a. Communicable disease: ....

   b. Hereditary diseases: ....

   c. Twin pregnancy/Bad obstetrical history: ....

3. Personal History:

   a. Dietary pattern: ....

   b. Sleeping pattern: ....

   c. Habits: ....

   d. Bowel elimination: ....

   e. Bladder elimination: ....

   f. Immunization history: ....

   g. Sexual history: ....

   h. Drugs history: .... Drug allergy: ....

4. Menstrual History: ....

5. Marital History: ....

6. Contraceptive History: ....

7. Previous Medical and Surgical History: ....

8. Previous Obstetrical History: ....

Sl No.	Year	Antenatal Period	Intranatal Period	Postnatal Period	Baby			Remarks
					Alive/Stillbirth	Sex	Weight (kg)	

9. Present Obstetrical History: ....

Antenatal period: ....

Intranatal period: ....

Postnatal period: ....

a. Physical Examination:
   - General condition:
   - General appearance:

     Body built: .... Health status: ....

     Activity: ....

     Head: .... Hair: ....
   - Facial appearance:

     Eyes: .... Ears: ....

     Nose: ....
   - Mouth:

     Gums: .... Teeth: ....

     Tongue: .... Tonsils: ....
   - Neck: ....

- Upper limbs:
- Chest: .... Lungs: ....

  Heart: ....
- Vital signs:

  Temperature: .... Pulse: ....

  Respiration: .... Blood pressure: ....

b. Obstetrical Examination:

- Breast:

  Size: .... Primary areola: ....

  Montgomery's tubercles: .... Secondary areola: ....

  Colostrums: .... Consistency: ....

  Discolorations: .... Any other: ....
- Uterus:

  Palpation: .... Fundal height: ....
- Bladder:

  Nipple protractility: .... Nodules/Lumps: ....
- Normal/Incontinence/Retention/Residual: ....
- Bowel sound: ....

  Bowel movement: ....

  Normal/Constipation/Loose Stool: ....
- Perineum:

  Condition: ....

  Intact/Laceration/Degree of Tear/Episiotomy: ....

  Assessment of Episiotomy/Tear: ....

  Lochia: .... Color: ....

  Rubra/Serosa/Alba Amount: ....

  Odor: ....
- Extremities:

  Range of joint movement: .... Pain: ....

  Discoloration: .... Any other: ....

ASSESSMENT OF THE NEWBORN

Name of the Baby: ....

Age of the Baby: .... Weight of the Baby: ....

Apgar Score: 1 Minute: .... 5 Minutes: ....

1. Anthropometric Measurement:

   Length: .... Weight: ....

   Head circumference: .... Chest circumference: ....

2. Vital Signs:

   Temperature: .... Heart rate: ....

   Respiration: ....

3. General Assessment:

   Activity: ....

   Head: ....

   Eyes: ....

   Ears: ....

   Mouth: ....

   Nose: ....

   Neck: ....

   Chest: ....

   Abdomen: ....

   Spine: ....

   Anus: ....

   Extremities: ....

4. Reflexes:

   Moro reflexes: ....

   Tonic neck reflexes: ....

   Feeding Reflexes: ....

   Rooting reflexes: .... Sucking reflexes: ....

   Swallowing reflexes: .... Gag reflexes: ....

   Blinking: ....

   Yawn: ....

   Protective Reflexes: ....

5. Elimination:

   Urine output: .... Cough and sneeze: ....

   Meconium: ....

NURSING CARE PLAN

Assessment	*Nursing Diagnosis*	*Goals*	*Nursing Intervention*	*Rationale*	*Nursing Implementation*	*Evaluation*

NURSING CARE PLAN

Assessment	*Nursing Diagnosis*	*Goals*	*Nursing Intervention*	*Rationale*	*Nursing Implementation*	*Evaluation*

NURSING CARE PLAN

Assessment	*Nursing Diagnosis*	*Goals*	*Nursing Intervention*	*Rationale*	*Nursing Implementation*	*Evaluation*

CLINICAL CHART OF PUERPERIUM

Date											
Temperature (°F)											*Fundal Height (cm)*
106											20
105											18
104											16
103											14
101											12
100											10
99											8
98											6
95											4
94											2
93											1
Pulse/mt											
BP (mm Hg)											
Respiration/mt											
Urine Output											
Bowel Examination											
Lochia											
Perineal Care											
Episiotomy Wound Healing											
Breastfeeding (Conditions of the Breast)											
Chief Complaints											
Treatment Given											

POSTNATAL EXAMINATION AND CARE (8)

Profile	*Mother*	*Father*
Name		
Age		
Educational status		
Occupation		
Religion		
Address		

OP/IP No.												
Date of admission												
EDD												
LMP												
Obstetrical score	G		P		L		A		S		D	
Weeks of gestation												
Date and time of delivery												
Type of delivery												
Sex of baby												
Weight of baby												
Postnatal day												
Date of discharge												

1. Socioeconomic Status:
   a. Total income of the family: ....
   b. Living standard:
   c. Type of the house:
      - Ownership of the House: ....
        Own/Rented: ....
        Number of rooms: ....
      - Environmental condition of the house:
        Lighting facility: ....
        Water facility: ....
        Drainage: ....
        Kitchen garden: ....
        Pet animals: ....

2. Family History:

Type of family: Nuclear Family/Joint Family

Sl No.	*Name of the Family Members*	*Age*	*Sex*	*Educational Status*	*Occupational Status*	*Relationship with the Mother*	*Health Status*
1.							
2.							
3.							
4.							
5.							
6.							
7.							
8.							
9.							

History of Any:

a. Communicable disease: ....

b. Hereditary diseases: ....

c. Twin pregnancy/Bad obstetrical history: ....

3. Personal History:

a. Dietary pattern: ....

b. Sleeping pattern: ....

c. Habits: ....

d. Bowel elimination: ....

e. Bladder elimination: ....

f. Immunization history: ....

g. Sexual history: ....

h. Drugs history: .... Drug allergy: ....

4. Menstrual History: ....

5. Marital History: ....

6. Contraceptive History: ....

7. Previous Medical and Surgical History: ....

8. Previous Obstetrical History: ....

Sl No.	*Year*	*Antenatal Period*	*Intranatal Period*	*Postnatal Period*	*Baby*			*Remarks*
					Alive/Stillbirth	*Sex*	*Weight (kg)*	

9. Present Obstetrical History: ....

Antenatal period: ....

Intranatal period: ....

Postnatal period: ....

a. Physical Examination:

- General condition:
- General appearance:

  Body built: .... Health status: ....

  Activity: ....

  Head: .... Hair: ....
- Facial appearance:

  Eyes: .... Ears: ....

  Nose: ....
- Mouth:

  Gums: .... Teeth: ....

  Tongue: .... Tonsils: ....
- Neck: ....

- Upper limbs:
- Chest: .... Lungs: ....
  Heart: ....
- Vital signs:
  Temperature: .... Pulse: ....
  Respiration: .... Blood pressure: ....

b. Obstetrical Examination:

- Breast:
  Size: .... Primary areola: ....
  Montgomery's tubercles: .... Secondary areola: ....
  Colostrums: .... Consistency: ....
  Discolorations: .... Any other: ....
- Uterus:
  Palpation: .... Fundal height: ....
- Bladder:
  Nipple protractility: .... Nodules/Lumps: ....
- Normal/Incontinence/Retention/Residual: ....
- Bowel sound: ....
  Bowel movement: ....
  Normal/Constipation/Loose Stool: ....
- Perineum:
  Condition: ....
  Intact/Laceration/Degree of Tear/Episiotomy: ....
  Assessment of Episiotomy/Tear: ....
  Lochia: .... Color: ....
  Rubra/Serosa/Alba Amount: ....
  Odor: ....
- Extremities:
  Range of joint movement: .... Pain: ....
  Discoloration: .... Any other: ....

ASSESSMENT OF THE NEWBORN

Name of the Baby: ....

Age of the Baby: .... Weight of the Baby: ....

Apgar Score: 1 Minute: .... 5 Minutes: ....

1. Anthropometric Measurement:

   Length: .... Weight: ....

   Head circumference: .... Chest circumference: ....

2. Vital Signs:

   Temperature: .... Heart rate: ....

   Respiration: ....

3. General Assessment:

   Activity: ....

   Head: ....

   Eyes: ....

   Ears: ....

   Mouth: ....

   Nose: ....

   Neck: ....

   Chest: ....

   Abdomen: ....

   Spine: ....

   Anus: ....

   Extremities: ....

4. Reflexes:

   Moro reflexes: ....

   Tonic neck reflexes: ....

   Feeding Reflexes: ....

   Rooting reflexes: .... Sucking reflexes: ....

   Swallowing reflexes: .... Gag reflexes: ....

   Blinking: ....

   Yawn: ....

   Protective Reflexes: ....

5. Elimination:

   Urine output: .... Cough and sneeze: ....

   Meconium: ....

NURSING CARE PLAN

Assessment	*Nursing Diagnosis*	*Goals*	*Nursing Intervention*	*Rationale*	*Nursing Implementation*	*Evaluation*

NURSING CARE PLAN

Assessment	*Nursing Diagnosis*	*Goals*	*Nursing Intervention*	*Rationale*	*Nursing Implementation*	*Evaluation*

NURSING CARE PLAN

Assessment	*Nursing Diagnosis*	*Goals*	*Nursing Intervention*	*Rationale*	*Nursing Implementation*	*Evaluation*

CLINICAL CHART OF PUERPERIUM

Date											
Temperature (°F)											*Fundal Height (cm)*
106											20
105											18
104											16
103											14
101											12
100											10
99											8
98											6
95											4
94											2
93											1
Pulse/mt											
BP (mm Hg)											
Respiration/mt											
Urine Output											
Bowel Examination											
Lochia											
Perineal Care											
Episiotomy Wound Healing											
Breastfeeding (Conditions of the Breast)											
Chief Complaints											
Treatment Given											

POSTNATAL EXAMINATION AND CARE (9)

Profile	*Mother*	*Father*
Name		
Age		
Educational status		
Occupation		
Religion		
Address		

OP/IP No.												
Date of admission												
EDD												
LMP												
Obstetrical score	G		P		L		A		S		D	
Weeks of gestation												
Date and time of delivery												
Type of delivery												
Sex of baby												
Weight of baby												
Postnatal day												
Date of discharge												

1. Socioeconomic Status:
   a. Total income of the family: ....
   b. Living standard:
   c. Type of the house:
      - Ownership of the House: ....
        Own/Rented: ....
        Number of rooms: ....
      - Environmental condition of the house:
        Lighting facility: ....
        Water facility: ....
        Drainage: ....
        Kitchen garden: ....
        Pet animals: ....

2. Family History:

   Type of family: Nuclear Family/Joint Family

Sl No.	*Name of the Family Members*	*Age*	*Sex*	*Educational Status*	*Occupational Status*	*Relationship with the Mother*	*Health Status*
1.							
2.							
3.							
4.							
5.							
6.							
7.							
8.							
9.							

   History of Any:

   a. Communicable disease: ....

   b. Hereditary diseases: ....

   c. Twin pregnancy/Bad obstetrical history: ....

3. Personal History:

   a. Dietary pattern: ....

   b. Sleeping pattern: ....

   c. Habits: ....

   d. Bowel elimination: ....

   e. Bladder elimination: ....

   f. Immunization history: ....

   g. Sexual history: ....

   h. Drugs history: .... Drug allergy: ....

4. Menstrual History: ....

5. Marital History: ....

6. Contraceptive History: ....

7. Previous Medical and Surgical History: ....

8. Previous Obstetrical History: ....

Sl No.	*Year*	*Antenatal Period*	*Intranatal Period*	*Postnatal Period*	*Baby*			*Remarks*
					Alive/Stillbirth	*Sex*	*Weight (kg)*	

9. Present Obstetrical History: ....

Antenatal period: ....

Intranatal period: ....

Postnatal period: ....

a. Physical Examination:

- General condition:
- General appearance:

  Body built: .... Health status: ....

  Activity: ....

  Head: .... Hair: ....

- Facial appearance:

  Eyes: .... Ears: ....

  Nose: ....

- Mouth:

  Gums: .... Teeth: ....

  Tongue: .... Tonsils: ....

- Neck: ....

- Upper limbs:
- Chest: .... Lungs: ....

  Heart: ....
- Vital signs:

  Temperature: .... Pulse: ....

  Respiration: .... Blood pressure: ....

b. Obstetrical Examination:

- Breast:

  Size: .... Primary areola: ....

  Montgomery's tubercles: .... Secondary areola: ....

  Colostrums: .... Consistency: ....

  Discolorations: .... Any other: ....
- Uterus:

  Palpation: .... Fundal height: ....
- Bladder:

  Nipple protractility: .... Nodules/Lumps: ....
- Normal/Incontinence/Retention/Residual: ....
- Bowel sound: ....

  Bowel movement: ....

  Normal/Constipation/Loose Stool: ....
- Perineum:

  Condition: ....

  Intact/Laceration/Degree of Tear/Episiotomy: ....

  Assessment of Episiotomy/Tear: ....

  Lochia: .... Color: ....

  Rubra/Serosa/Alba Amount: ....

  Odor: ....
- Extremities:

  Range of joint movement: .... Pain: ....

  Discoloration: .... Any other: ....

ASSESSMENT OF THE NEWBORN

Name of the Baby: ....

Age of the Baby: .... Weight of the Baby: ....

Apgar Score: 1 Minute: .... 5 Minutes: ....

1. Anthropometric Measurement:

   Length: .... Weight: ....

   Head circumference: .... Chest circumference: ....

2. Vital Signs:

   Temperature: .... Heart rate: ....

   Respiration: ....

3. General Assessment:

   Activity: ....

   Head: ....

   Eyes: ....

   Ears: ....

   Mouth: ....

   Nose: ....

   Neck: ....

   Chest: ....

   Abdomen: ....

   Spine: ....

   Anus: ....

   Extremities: ....

4. Reflexes:

   Moro reflexes: ....

   Tonic neck reflexes: ....

   Feeding Reflexes: ....

   Rooting reflexes: .... Sucking reflexes: ....

   Swallowing reflexes: .... Gag reflexes: ....

   Blinking: ....

   Yawn: ....

   Protective Reflexes: ....

5. Elimination:

   Urine output: .... Cough and sneeze: ....

   Meconium: ....

NURSING CARE PLAN

Assessment	*Nursing Diagnosis*	*Goals*	*Nursing Intervention*	*Rationale*	*Nursing Implementation*	*Evaluation*

NURSING CARE PLAN

Assessment	*Nursing Diagnosis*	*Goals*	*Nursing Intervention*	*Rationale*	*Nursing Implementation*	*Evaluation*

NURSING CARE PLAN

Assessment	*Nursing Diagnosis*	*Goals*	*Nursing Intervention*	*Rationale*	*Nursing Implementation*	*Evaluation*

CLINICAL CHART OF PUERPERIUM

Date											
Temperature (°F)											*Fundal Height (cm)*
106											20
105											18
104											16
103											14
101											12
100											10
99											8
98											6
95											4
94											2
93											1
Pulse/mt											
BP (mm Hg)											
Respiration/mt											
Urine Output											
Bowel Examination											
Lochia											
Perineal Care											
Episiotomy Wound Healing											
Breastfeeding (Conditions of the Breast)											
Chief Complaints											
Treatment Given											

POSTNATAL EXAMINATION AND CARE (10)

Profile	*Mother*	*Father*
Name		
Age		
Educational status		
Occupation		
Religion		
Address		

OP/IP No.												
Date of admission												
EDD												
LMP												
Obstetrical score	G		P		L		A		S		D	
Weeks of gestation												
Date and time of delivery												
Type of delivery												
Sex of baby												
Weight of baby												
Postnatal day												
Date of discharge												

1. Socioeconomic Status:
   a. Total income of the family: ....
   b. Living standard:
   c. Type of the house:
      - Ownership of the House: ....

        Own/Rented: ....

        Number of rooms: ....
      - Environmental condition of the house:

        Lighting facility: ....

        Water facility: ....

        Drainage: ....

        Kitchen garden: ....

        Pet animals: ....

2. Family History:

   Type of family: Nuclear Family/Joint Family

Sl No.	*Name of the Family Members*	*Age*	*Sex*	*Educational Status*	*Occupational Status*	*Relationship with the Mother*	*Health Status*
1.							
2.							
3.							
4.							
5.							
6.							
7.							
8.							
9.							

   History of Any:

   a. Communicable disease: ....

   b. Hereditary diseases: ....

   c. Twin pregnancy/Bad obstetrical history: ....

3. Personal History:

   a. Dietary pattern: ....

   b. Sleeping pattern: ....

   c. Habits: ....

   d. Bowel elimination: ....

   e. Bladder elimination: ....

   f. Immunization history: ....

   g. Sexual history: ....

   h. Drugs history: .... Drug allergy: ....

4. Menstrual History: ....

5. Marital History: ....

6. Contraceptive History: ....

7. Previous Medical and Surgical History: ....

8. Previous Obstetrical History: ....

Sl No.	Year	Antenatal Period	Intranatal Period	Postnatal Period	Baby			Remarks
					Alive/Stillbirth	Sex	Weight (kg)	

9. Present Obstetrical History: ....

Antenatal period: ....

Intranatal period: ....

Postnatal period: ....

a. Physical Examination:

- General condition:
- General appearance:

  Body built: .... Health status: ....

  Activity: ....

  Head: .... Hair: ....
- Facial appearance:

  Eyes: .... Ears: ....

  Nose: ....
- Mouth:

  Gums: .... Teeth: ....

  Tongue: .... Tonsils: ....
- Neck: ....

- Upper limbs:
- Chest: .... Lungs: ....

  Heart: ....
- Vital signs:

  Temperature: .... Pulse: ....

  Respiration: .... Blood pressure: ....

b. Obstetrical Examination:

- Breast:

  Size: .... Primary areola: ....

  Montgomery's tubercles: .... Secondary areola: ....

  Colostrums: .... Consistency: ....

  Discolorations: .... Any other: ....
- Uterus:

  Palpation: .... Fundal height: ....
- Bladder:

  Nipple protractility: .... Nodules/Lumps: ....
- Normal/Incontinence/Retention/Residual: ....
- Bowel sound: ....

  Bowel movement: ....

  Normal/Constipation/Loose Stool: ....
- Perineum:

  Condition: ....

  Intact/Laceration/Degree of Tear/Episiotomy: ....

  Assessment of Episiotomy/Tear: ....

  Lochia: .... Color: ....

  Rubra/Serosa/Alba Amount: ....

  Odor: ....
- Extremities:

  Range of joint movement: .... Pain: ....

  Discoloration: .... Any other: ....

ASSESSMENT OF THE NEWBORN

Name of the Baby: ....

Age of the Baby: .... Weight of the Baby: ....

Apgar Score: 1 Minute: .... 5 Minutes: ....

1. Anthropometric Measurement:

   Length: .... Weight: ....

   Head circumference: .... Chest circumference: ....

2. Vital Signs:

   Temperature: .... Heart rate: ....

   Respiration: ....

3. General Assessment:

   Activity: ....

   Head: ....

   Eyes: ....

   Ears: ....

   Mouth: ....

   Nose: ....

   Neck: ....

   Chest: ....

   Abdomen: ....

   Spine: ....

   Anus: ....

   Extremities: ....

4. Reflexes:

   Moro reflexes: ....

   Tonic neck reflexes: ....

   Feeding Reflexes: ....

   Rooting reflexes: .... Sucking reflexes: ....

   Swallowing reflexes: .... Gag reflexes: ....

   Blinking: ....

   Yawn: ....

   Protective Reflexes: ....

5. Elimination:

   Urine output: .... Cough and sneeze: ....

   Meconium: ....

NURSING CARE PLAN

Assessment	*Nursing Diagnosis*	*Goals*	*Nursing Intervention*	*Rationale*	*Nursing Implementation*	*Evaluation*

NURSING CARE PLAN

Assessment	*Nursing Diagnosis*	*Goals*	*Nursing Intervention*	*Rationale*	*Nursing Implementation*	*Evaluation*

NURSING CARE PLAN

Assessment	*Nursing Diagnosis*	*Goals*	*Nursing Intervention*	*Rationale*	*Nursing Implementation*	*Evaluation*

CLINICAL CHART OF PUERPERIUM

Date											
Temperature (°F)											*Fundal Height (cm)*
106											20
105											18
104											16
103											14
101											12
100											10
99											8
98											6
95											4
94											2
93											1
Pulse/mt											
BP (mm Hg)											
Respiration/mt											
Urine Output											
Bowel Examination											
Lochia											
Perineal Care											
Episiotomy Wound Healing											
Breastfeeding (Conditions of the Breast)											
Chief Complaints											
Treatment Given											

POSTNATAL EXAMINATION AND CARE (11)

Profile	*Mother*	*Father*
Name		
Age		
Educational status		
Occupation		
Religion		
Address		

OP/IP No.												
Date of admission												
EDD												
LMP												
Obstetrical score	G		P		L		A		S		D	
Weeks of gestation												
Date and time of delivery												
Type of delivery												
Sex of baby												
Weight of baby												
Postnatal day												
Date of discharge												

1. Socioeconomic Status:
   a. Total income of the family: ....
   b. Living standard:
   c. Type of the house:
      - Ownership of the House: ....
        Own/Rented: ....
        Number of rooms: ....
      - Environmental condition of the house:
        Lighting facility: ....
        Water facility: ....
        Drainage: ....
        Kitchen garden: ....
        Pet animals: ....

2. Family History:

   Type of family: Nuclear Family/Joint Family

Sl No.	*Name of the Family Members*	*Age*	*Sex*	*Educational Status*	*Occupational Status*	*Relationship with the Mother*	*Health Status*
1.							
2.							
3.							
4.							
5.							
6.							
7.							
8.							
9.							

   History of Any:

   a. Communicable disease: ....

   b. Hereditary diseases: ....

   c. Twin pregnancy/Bad obstetrical history: ....

3. Personal History:

   a. Dietary pattern: ....

   b. Sleeping pattern: ....

   c. Habits: ....

   d. Bowel elimination: ....

   e. Bladder elimination: ....

   f. Immunization history: ....

   g. Sexual history: ....

   h. Drugs history: .... Drug allergy: ....

4. Menstrual History: ....

5. Marital History: ....

6. Contraceptive History: ....

7. Previous Medical and Surgical History: ....

8. Previous Obstetrical History: ....

Sl No.	*Year*	*Antenatal Period*	*Intranatal Period*	*Postnatal Period*	*Baby*			*Remarks*
					Alive/Stillbirth	*Sex*	*Weight (kg)*	

9. Present Obstetrical History: ....

Antenatal period: ....

Intranatal period: ....

Postnatal period: ....

a. Physical Examination:

- General condition:
- General appearance:

Body built: .... Health status: ....

Activity: ....

Head: .... Hair: ....

- Facial appearance:

Eyes: .... Ears: ....

Nose: ....

- Mouth:

Gums: .... Teeth: ....

Tongue: .... Tonsils: ....

- Neck: ....

- Upper limbs:
- Chest: .... Lungs: ....

  Heart: ....
- Vital signs:

  Temperature: .... Pulse: ....

  Respiration: .... Blood pressure: ....

b. Obstetrical Examination:

- Breast:

  Size: .... Primary areola: ....

  Montgomery's tubercles: .... Secondary areola: ....

  Colostrums: .... Consistency: ....

  Discolorations: .... Any other: ....
- Uterus:

  Palpation: .... Fundal height: ....
- Bladder:

  Nipple protractility: .... Nodules/Lumps: ....
- Normal/Incontinence/Retention/Residual: ....
- Bowel sound: ....

  Bowel movement: ....

  Normal/Constipation/Loose Stool: ....
- Perineum:

  Condition: ....

  Intact/Laceration/Degree of Tear/Episiotomy: ....

  Assessment of Episiotomy/Tear: ....

  Lochia: .... Color: ....

  Rubra/Serosa/Alba Amount: ....

  Odor: ....
- Extremities:

  Range of joint movement: .... Pain: ....

  Discoloration: .... Any other: ....

ASSESSMENT OF THE NEWBORN

Name of the Baby: ....

Age of the Baby: .... Weight of the Baby: ....

Apgar Score: 1 Minute: .... 5 Minutes: ....

1. Anthropometric Measurement:

   Length: .... Weight: ....

   Head circumference: .... Chest circumference: ....

2. Vital Signs:

   Temperature: .... Heart rate: ....

   Respiration: ....

3. General Assessment:

   Activity: ....

   Head: ....

   Eyes: ....

   Ears: ....

   Mouth: ....

   Nose: ....

   Neck: ....

   Chest: ....

   Abdomen: ....

   Spine: ....

   Anus: ....

   Extremities: ....

4. Reflexes:

   Moro reflexes: ....

   Tonic neck reflexes: ....

   Feeding Reflexes: ....

   Rooting reflexes: .... Sucking reflexes: ....

   Swallowing reflexes: .... Gag reflexes: ....

   Blinking: ....

   Yawn: ....

   Protective Reflexes: ....

5. Elimination:

   Urine output: .... Cough and sneeze: ....

   Meconium: ....

NURSING CARE PLAN

Assessment	*Nursing Diagnosis*	*Goals*	*Nursing Intervention*	*Rationale*	*Nursing Implementation*	*Evaluation*

NURSING CARE PLAN

Assessment	*Nursing Diagnosis*	*Goals*	*Nursing Intervention*	*Rationale*	*Nursing Implementation*	*Evaluation*

NURSING CARE PLAN

Assessment	*Nursing Diagnosis*	*Goals*	*Nursing Intervention*	*Rationale*	*Nursing Implementation*	*Evaluation*

CLINICAL CHART OF PUERPERIUM

Date											
Temperature (°F)											*Fundal Height (cm)*
106											20
105											18
104											16
103											14
101											12
100											10
99											8
98											6
95											4
94											2
93											1
Pulse/mt											
BP (mm Hg)											
Respiration/mt											
Urine Output											
Bowel Examination											
Lochia											
Perineal Care											
Episiotomy Wound Healing											
Breastfeeding (Conditions of the Breast)											
Chief Complaints											
Treatment Given											

POSTNATAL EXAMINATION AND CARE (12)

Profile	*Mother*	*Father*
Name		
Age		
Educational status		
Occupation		
Religion		
Address		

OP/IP No.												
Date of admission												
EDD												
LMP												
Obstetrical score	G		P		L		A		S		D	
Weeks of gestation												
Date and time of delivery												
Type of delivery												
Sex of baby												
Weight of baby												
Postnatal day												
Date of discharge												

1. Socioeconomic Status:
   a. Total income of the family: ....
   b. Living standard:
   c. Type of the house:
      - Ownership of the House: ....
        Own/Rented: ....
        Number of rooms: ....
      - Environmental condition of the house:
        Lighting facility: ....
        Water facility: ....
        Drainage: ....
        Kitchen garden: ....
        Pet animals: ....

2. Family History:

   Type of family: Nuclear Family/Joint Family

Sl No.	*Name of the Family Members*	*Age*	*Sex*	*Educational Status*	*Occupational Status*	*Relationship with the Mother*	*Health Status*
1.							
2.							
3.							
4.							
5.							
6.							
7.							
8.							
9.							

   History of Any:

   a. Communicable disease: ....

   b. Hereditary diseases: ....

   c. Twin pregnancy/Bad obstetrical history: ....

3. Personal History:

   a. Dietary pattern: ....

   b. Sleeping pattern: ....

   c. Habits: ....

   d. Bowel elimination: ....

   e. Bladder elimination: ....

   f. Immunization history: ....

   g. Sexual history: ....

   h. Drugs history: .... Drug allergy: ....

4. Menstrual History: ....

5. Marital History: ....

6. Contraceptive History: ....

7. Previous Medical and Surgical History: ....

8. Previous Obstetrical History: ....

Sl No.	*Year*	*Antenatal Period*	*Intranatal Period*	*Postnatal Period*	*Baby*			*Remarks*
					Alive/Stillbirth	*Sex*	*Weight (kg)*	

9. Present Obstetrical History: ....

Antenatal period: ....

Intranatal period: ....

Postnatal period: ....

a. Physical Examination:

- General condition:
- General appearance:

  Body built: .... Health status: ....

  Activity: ....

  Head: .... Hair: ....
- Facial appearance:

  Eyes: .... Ears: ....

  Nose: ....
- Mouth:

  Gums: .... Teeth: ....

  Tongue: .... Tonsils: ....
- Neck: ....

- Upper limbs:
- Chest: .... Lungs: ....

  Heart: ....
- Vital signs:

  Temperature: .... Pulse: ....

  Respiration: .... Blood pressure: ....

b. Obstetrical Examination:

- Breast:

  Size: .... Primary areola: ....

  Montgomery's tubercles: .... Secondary areola: ....

  Colostrums: .... Consistency: ....

  Discolorations: .... Any other: ....
- Uterus:

  Palpation: .... Fundal height: ....
- Bladder:

  Nipple protractility: .... Nodules/Lumps: ....
- Normal/Incontinence/Retention/Residual: ....
- Bowel sound: ....

  Bowel movement: ....

  Normal/Constipation/Loose Stool: ....
- Perineum:

  Condition: ....

  Intact/Laceration/Degree of Tear/Episiotomy: ....

  Assessment of Episiotomy/Tear: ....

  Lochia: .... Color: ....

  Rubra/Serosa/Alba Amount: ....

  Odor: ....
- Extremities:

  Range of joint movement: .... Pain: ....

  Discoloration: .... Any other: ....

ASSESSMENT OF THE NEWBORN

Name of the Baby: ....

Age of the Baby: .... Weight of the Baby: ....

Apgar Score: 1 Minute: .... 5 Minutes: ....

1. Anthropometric Measurement:

   Length: .... Weight: ....

   Head circumference: .... Chest circumference: ....

2. Vital Signs:

   Temperature: .... Heart rate: ....

   Respiration: ....

3. General Assessment:

   Activity: ....

   Head: ....

   Eyes: ....

   Ears: ....

   Mouth: ....

   Nose: ....

   Neck: ....

   Chest: ....

   Abdomen: ....

   Spine: ....

   Anus: ....

   Extremities: ....

4. Reflexes:

   Moro reflexes: ....

   Tonic neck reflexes: ....

   Feeding Reflexes: ....

   Rooting reflexes: .... Sucking reflexes: ....

   Swallowing reflexes: .... Gag reflexes: ....

   Blinking: ....

   Yawn: ....

   Protective Reflexes: ....

5. Elimination:

   Urine output: .... Cough and sneeze: ....

   Meconium: ....

NURSING CARE PLAN

Assessment	*Nursing Diagnosis*	*Goals*	*Nursing Intervention*	*Rationale*	*Nursing Implementation*	*Evaluation*

NURSING CARE PLAN

Assessment	*Nursing Diagnosis*	*Goals*	*Nursing Intervention*	*Rationale*	*Nursing Implementation*	*Evaluation*

NURSING CARE PLAN

Assessment	*Nursing Diagnosis*	*Goals*	*Nursing Intervention*	*Rationale*	*Nursing Implementation*	*Evaluation*

CLINICAL CHART OF PUERPERIUM

Date											
Temperature (°F)											*Fundal Height (cm)*
106											20
105											18
104											16
103											14
101											12
100											10
99											8
98											6
95											4
94											2
93											1
Pulse/mt											
BP (mm Hg)											
Respiration/mt											
Urine Output											
Bowel Examination											
Lochia											
Perineal Care											
Episiotomy Wound Healing											
Breastfeeding (Conditions of the Breast)											
Chief Complaints											
Treatment Given											

POSTNATAL EXAMINATION AND CARE (13)

Profile	*Mother*	*Father*
Name		
Age		
Educational status		
Occupation		
Religion		
Address		

OP/IP No.												
Date of admission												
EDD												
LMP												
Obstetrical score	G		P		L		A		S		D	
Weeks of gestation												
Date and time of delivery												
Type of delivery												
Sex of baby												
Weight of baby												
Postnatal day												
Date of discharge												

1. Socioeconomic Status:
   a. Total income of the family: ....
   b. Living standard:
   c. Type of the house:
      - Ownership of the House: ....
        Own/Rented: ....
        Number of rooms: ....
      - Environmental condition of the house:
        Lighting facility: ....
        Water facility: ....
        Drainage: ....
        Kitchen garden: ....
        Pet animals: ....

2. Family History:

Type of family: Nuclear Family/Joint Family

Sl No.	*Name of the Family Members*	*Age*	*Sex*	*Educational Status*	*Occupational Status*	*Relationship with the Mother*	*Health Status*
1.							
2.							
3.							
4.							
5.							
6.							
7.							
8.							
9.							

History of Any:

a. Communicable disease: ....

b. Hereditary diseases: ....

c. Twin pregnancy/Bad obstetrical history: ....

3. Personal History:

a. Dietary pattern: ....

b. Sleeping pattern: ....

c. Habits: ....

d. Bowel elimination: ....

e. Bladder elimination: ....

f. Immunization history: ....

g. Sexual history: ....

h. Drugs history: .... Drug allergy: ....

4. Menstrual History: ....

5. Marital History: ....

6. Contraceptive History: ....

7. Previous Medical and Surgical History: ....

8. Previous Obstetrical History: ....

Sl No.	Year	Antenatal Period	Intranatal Period	Postnatal Period	Baby			Remarks
					Alive/Stillbirth	Sex	Weight (kg)	

9. Present Obstetrical History: ....

Antenatal period: ....

Intranatal period: ....

Postnatal period: ....

a. Physical Examination:

- General condition:
- General appearance:

  Body built: .... Health status: ....

  Activity: ....

  Head: .... Hair: ....
- Facial appearance:

  Eyes: .... Ears: ....

  Nose: ....
- Mouth:

  Gums: .... Teeth: ....

  Tongue: .... Tonsils: ....
- Neck: ....

- Upper limbs:
- Chest: .... Lungs: ....

  Heart: ....
- Vital signs:

  Temperature: .... Pulse: ....

  Respiration: .... Blood pressure: ....

b. Obstetrical Examination:

- Breast:

  Size: .... Primary areola: ....

  Montgomery's tubercles: .... Secondary areola: ....

  Colostrums: .... Consistency: ....

  Discolorations: .... Any other: ....
- Uterus:

  Palpation: .... Fundal height: ....
- Bladder:

  Nipple protractility: .... Nodules/Lumps: ....
- Normal/Incontinence/Retention/Residual: ....
- Bowel sound: ....

  Bowel movement: ....

  Normal/Constipation/Loose Stool: ....
- Perineum:

  Condition: ....

  Intact/Laceration/Degree of Tear/Episiotomy: ....

  Assessment of Episiotomy/Tear: ....

  Lochia: .... Color: ....

  Rubra/Serosa/Alba Amount: ....

  Odor: ....
- Extremities:

  Range of joint movement: .... Pain: ....

  Discoloration: .... Any other: ....

ASSESSMENT OF THE NEWBORN

Name of the Baby: ....

Age of the Baby: .... Weight of the Baby: ....

Apgar Score: 1 Minute: .... 5 Minutes: ....

1. Anthropometric Measurement:

   Length: .... Weight: ....

   Head circumference: .... Chest circumference: ....

2. Vital Signs:

   Temperature: .... Heart rate: ....

   Respiration: ....

3. General Assessment:

   Activity: ....

   Head: ....

   Eyes: ....

   Ears: ....

   Mouth: ....

   Nose: ....

   Neck: ....

   Chest: ....

   Abdomen: ....

   Spine: ....

   Anus: ....

   Extremities: ....

4. Reflexes:

   Moro reflexes: ....

   Tonic neck reflexes: ....

   Feeding Reflexes: ....

   Rooting reflexes: .... Sucking reflexes: ....

   Swallowing reflexes: .... Gag reflexes: ....

   Blinking: ....

   Yawn: ....

   Protective Reflexes: ....

5. Elimination:

   Urine output: .... Cough and sneeze: ....

   Meconium: ....

NURSING CARE PLAN

Assessment	*Nursing Diagnosis*	*Goals*	*Nursing Intervention*	*Rationale*	*Nursing Implementation*	*Evaluation*

NURSING CARE PLAN

Assessment	*Nursing Diagnosis*	*Goals*	*Nursing Intervention*	*Rationale*	*Nursing Implementation*	*Evaluation*

NURSING CARE PLAN

Assessment	*Nursing Diagnosis*	*Goals*	*Nursing Intervention*	*Rationale*	*Nursing Implementation*	*Evaluation*

CLINICAL CHART OF PUERPERIUM

Date											
Temperature (°F)											*Fundal Height (cm)*
106											20
105											18
104											16
103											14
101											12
100											10
99											8
98											6
95											4
94											2
93											1
Pulse/mt											
BP (mm Hg)											
Respiration/mt											
Urine Output											
Bowel Examination											
Lochia											
Perineal Care											
Episiotomy Wound Healing											
Breastfeeding (Conditions of the Breast)											
Chief Complaints											
Treatment Given											

POSTNATAL EXAMINATION AND CARE (14)

Profile	*Mother*	*Father*
Name		
Age		
Educational status		
Occupation		
Religion		
Address		

OP/IP No.												
Date of admission												
EDD												
LMP												
Obstetrical score	G		P		L		A		S		D	
Weeks of gestation												
Date and time of delivery												
Type of delivery												
Sex of baby												
Weight of baby												
Postnatal day												
Date of discharge												

1. Socioeconomic Status:
   a. Total income of the family: ....
   b. Living standard:
   c. Type of the house:
      - Ownership of the House: ....
        Own/Rented: ....
        Number of rooms: ....
      - Environmental condition of the house:
        Lighting facility: ....
        Water facility: ....
        Drainage: ....
        Kitchen garden: ....
        Pet animals: ....

2. Family History:

   Type of family: Nuclear Family/Joint Family

Sl No.	*Name of the Family Members*	*Age*	*Sex*	*Educational Status*	*Occupational Status*	*Relationship with the Mother*	*Health Status*
1.							
2.							
3.							
4.							
5.							
6.							
7.							
8.							
9.							

   History of Any:

   a. Communicable disease: ....

   b. Hereditary diseases: ....

   c. Twin pregnancy/Bad obstetrical history: ....

3. Personal History:

   a. Dietary pattern: ....

   b. Sleeping pattern: ....

   c. Habits: ....

   d. Bowel elimination: ....

   e. Bladder elimination: ....

   f. Immunization history: ....

   g. Sexual history: ....

   h. Drugs history: .... Drug allergy: ....

4. Menstrual History: ....

5. Marital History: ....

6. Contraceptive History: ....

7. Previous Medical and Surgical History: ....

8. Previous Obstetrical History: ....

Sl No.	*Year*	*Antenatal Period*	*Intranatal Period*	*Postnatal Period*	*Baby*			*Remarks*
					Alive/Stillbirth	*Sex*	*Weight (kg)*	

9. Present Obstetrical History: ....

Antenatal period: ....

Intranatal period: ....

Postnatal period: ....

a. Physical Examination:

- General condition:
- General appearance:

  Body built: .... Health status: ....

  Activity: ....

  Head: .... Hair: ....
- Facial appearance:

  Eyes: .... Ears: ....

  Nose: ....
- Mouth:

  Gums: .... Teeth: ....

  Tongue: .... Tonsils: ....
- Neck: ....

- Upper limbs:
- Chest: .... Lungs: ....

  Heart: ....
- Vital signs:

  Temperature: .... Pulse: ....

  Respiration: .... Blood pressure: ....

b. Obstetrical Examination:

- Breast:

  Size: .... Primary areola: ....

  Montgomery's tubercles: .... Secondary areola: ....

  Colostrums: .... Consistency: ....

  Discolorations: .... Any other: ....
- Uterus:

  Palpation: .... Fundal height: ....
- Bladder:

  Nipple protractility: .... Nodules/Lumps: ....
- Normal/Incontinence/Retention/Residual: ....
- Bowel sound: ....

  Bowel movement: ....

  Normal/Constipation/Loose Stool: ....
- Perineum:

  Condition: ....

  Intact/Laceration/Degree of Tear/Episiotomy: ....

  Assessment of Episiotomy/Tear: ....

  Lochia: .... Color: ....

  Rubra/Serosa/Alba Amount: ....

  Odor: ....
- Extremities:

  Range of joint movement: .... Pain: ....

  Discoloration: .... Any other: ....

ASSESSMENT OF THE NEWBORN

Name of the Baby: ....

Age of the Baby: .... Weight of the Baby: ....

Apgar Score: 1 Minute: .... 5 Minutes: ....

1. Anthropometric Measurement:

   Length: .... Weight: ....

   Head circumference: .... Chest circumference: ....

2. Vital Signs:

   Temperature: .... Heart rate: ....

   Respiration: ....

3. General Assessment:

   Activity: ....

   Head: ....

   Eyes: ....

   Ears: ....

   Mouth: ....

   Nose: ....

   Neck: ....

   Chest: ....

   Abdomen: ....

   Spine: ....

   Anus: ....

   Extremities: ....

4. Reflexes:

   Moro reflexes: ....

   Tonic neck reflexes: ....

   Feeding Reflexes: ....

   Rooting reflexes: .... Sucking reflexes: ....

   Swallowing reflexes: .... Gag reflexes: ....

   Blinking: ....

   Yawn: ....

   Protective Reflexes: ....

5. Elimination:

   Urine output: .... Cough and sneeze: ....

   Meconium: ....

NURSING CARE PLAN

Assessment	*Nursing Diagnosis*	*Goals*	*Nursing Intervention*	*Rationale*	*Nursing Implementation*	*Evaluation*

NURSING CARE PLAN

Assessment	Nursing Diagnosis	Goals	Nursing Intervention	Rationale	Nursing Implementation	Evaluation

NURSING CARE PLAN

Assessment	*Nursing Diagnosis*	*Goals*	*Nursing Intervention*	*Rationale*	*Nursing Implementation*	*Evaluation*

CLINICAL CHART OF PUERPERIUM

Date											
Temperature (°F)											*Fundal Height (cm)*
106											20
105											18
104											16
103											14
101											12
100											10
99											8
98											6
95											4
94											2
93											1
Pulse/mt											
BP (mm Hg)											
Respiration/mt											
Urine Output											
Bowel Examination											
Lochia											
Perineal Care											
Episiotomy Wound Healing											
Breastfeeding (Conditions of the Breast)											
Chief Complaints											
Treatment Given											

POSTNATAL EXAMINATION AND CARE (15)

Profile	*Mother*	*Father*
Name		
Age		
Educational status		
Occupation		
Religion		
Address		

OP/IP No.												
Date of admission												
EDD												
LMP												
Obstetrical score	G		P		L		A		S		D	
Weeks of gestation												
Date and time of delivery												
Type of delivery												
Sex of baby												
Weight of baby												
Postnatal day												
Date of discharge												

1. Socioeconomic Status:
   a. Total income of the family: ....
   b. Living standard:
   c. Type of the house:
      - Ownership of the House: ....
        Own/Rented: ....
        Number of rooms: ....
      - Environmental condition of the house:
        Lighting facility: ....
        Water facility: ....
        Drainage: ....
        Kitchen garden: ....
        Pet animals: ....

2. Family History:

   Type of family: Nuclear Family/Joint Family

Sl No.	*Name of the Family Members*	*Age*	*Sex*	*Educational Status*	*Occupational Status*	*Relationship with the Mother*	*Health Status*
1.							
2.							
3.							
4.							
5.							
6.							
7.							
8.							
9.							

   History of Any:

   a. Communicable disease: ....

   b. Hereditary diseases: ....

   c. Twin pregnancy/Bad obstetrical history: ....

3. Personal History:

   a. Dietary pattern: ....

   b. Sleeping pattern: ....

   c. Habits: ....

   d. Bowel elimination: ....

   e. Bladder elimination: ....

   f. Immunization history: ....

   g. Sexual history: ....

   h. Drugs history: .... Drug allergy: ....

4. Menstrual History: ....

5. Marital History: ....

6. Contraceptive History: ....

7. Previous Medical and Surgical History: ....

8. Previous Obstetrical History: ....

Sl No.	Year	Antenatal Period	Intranatal Period	Postnatal Period	Baby			Remarks
					Alive/Stillbirth	Sex	Weight (kg)	

9. Present Obstetrical History: ....

Antenatal period: ....

Intranatal period: ....

Postnatal period: ....

a. Physical Examination:

- General condition:
- General appearance:

  Body built: .... Health status: ....

  Activity: ....

  Head: .... Hair: ....
- Facial appearance:

  Eyes: .... Ears: ....

  Nose: ....
- Mouth:

  Gums: .... Teeth: ....

  Tongue: .... Tonsils: ....
- Neck: ....

- Upper limbs:
- Chest: .... Lungs: ....

  Heart: ....
- Vital signs:

  Temperature: .... Pulse: ....

  Respiration: .... Blood pressure: ....

b. Obstetrical Examination:

- Breast:

  Size: .... Primary areola: ....

  Montgomery's tubercles: .... Secondary areola: ....

  Colostrums: .... Consistency: ....

  Discolorations: .... Any other: ....
- Uterus:

  Palpation: .... Fundal height: ....
- Bladder:

  Nipple protractility: .... Nodules/Lumps: ....
- Normal/Incontinence/Retention/Residual: ....
- Bowel sound: ....

  Bowel movement: ....

  Normal/Constipation/Loose Stool: ....
- Perineum:

  Condition: ....

  Intact/Laceration/Degree of Tear/Episiotomy: ....

  Assessment of Episiotomy/Tear: ....

  Lochia: .... Color: ....

  Rubra/Serosa/Alba Amount: ....

  Odor: ....
- Extremities:

  Range of joint movement: .... Pain: ....

  Discoloration: .... Any other: ....

ASSESSMENT OF THE NEWBORN

Name of the Baby: ....

Age of the Baby: .... Weight of the Baby: ....

Apgar Score: 1 Minute: .... 5 Minutes: ....

1. Anthropometric Measurement:
   Length: .... Weight: ....
   Head circumference: .... Chest circumference: ....
2. Vital Signs:
   Temperature: .... Heart rate: ....
   Respiration: ....
3. General Assessment:
   Activity: ....
   Head: ....
   Eyes: ....
   Ears: ....
   Mouth: ....
   Nose: ....
   Neck: ....
   Chest: ....
   Abdomen: ....
   Spine: ....
   Anus: ....
   Extremities: ....
4. Reflexes:
   Moro reflexes: ....
   Tonic neck reflexes: ....
   Feeding Reflexes: ....
   Rooting reflexes: .... Sucking reflexes: ....
   Swallowing reflexes: .... Gag reflexes: ....
   Blinking: ....
   Yawn: ....
   Protective Reflexes: ....
5. Elimination:
   Urine output: .... Cough and sneeze: ....
   Meconium: ....

NURSING CARE PLAN

Assessment	*Nursing Diagnosis*	*Goals*	*Nursing Intervention*	*Rationale*	*Nursing Implementation*	*Evaluation*

NURSING CARE PLAN

Assessment	*Nursing Diagnosis*	*Goals*	*Nursing Intervention*	*Rationale*	*Nursing Implementation*	*Evaluation*

NURSING CARE PLAN

Assessment	*Nursing Diagnosis*	*Goals*	*Nursing Intervention*	*Rationale*	*Nursing Implementation*	*Evaluation*

CLINICAL CHART OF PUERPERIUM

Date											
Temperature (°F)											*Fundal Height (cm)*
106											20
105											18
104											16
103											14
101											12
100											10
99											8
98											6
95											4
94											2
93											1
Pulse/mt											
BP (mm Hg)											
Respiration/mt											
Urine Output											
Bowel Examination											
Lochia											
Perineal Care											
Episiotomy Wound Healing											
Breastfeeding (Conditions of the Breast)											
Chief Complaints											
Treatment Given											

CHAPTER 7

Neonatal Assessment and Care

NEONATAL EXAMINATION AND CARE/INCLUDING HIGH-RISK NEWBORN

Sl No.	*IP No.*	*Name of the Baby*	*Date and Time of Delivery*	*Type of Delivery*	*Condition of the Baby at Birth*			*Normal Neonate or High-risk Neonate*	*Delivery Conducted by*	*Date of Care Started*	*Date of Care Ended*	*Condition of the Baby at the Time of Discharge*
					Weight	*Sex*	*Apgar Score*					
1.												
2.												
3.												
4.												
5.												

Signature of the Supervisor

ASSESSMENT AND CARE OF THE NEWBORN (1)

1. Profile of the Newborn:

Name: ....

Name of the Hospital: ....

Inpatient (IP) Number (No): .... Ward: ....

Mother's Name: ....

Father's Name: ....

Address: ....

Date of Birth: .... Sex: Male/Female: ....

Birth Order: ....

Apgar Score:

1 minute: .... 5 minutes: ....

Religion: ....

Educational Status:

Mother: .... Father: ....

Occupation:

Father: .... Mother: ....

Total income of the family: ....

2. Birth History:

   a. Antenatal history:

      Age of mother: ....

      Type of marriage:

      Consanguineous: .... Nonconsanguineous: ....

      Degree of consanguinity: ....

      Antenatal checkups:

      Regular: .... Irregular: ....

      Tetanus toxoid:

      Yes/No: .... No. of doses: ....

      Any exposure to drug/radiation: ....

      If Yes: Specify: ....

      Any illness during pregnancy: ....

b. Intranatal History:

Date and time of delivery: ....

Place of delivery: ....

Delivery conducted by: ....

Mode of delivery: ....

Gestational age (in weeks): ....

Birth weight: .... kg

Cried at birth: Yes/No: ....

Apgar score: 1 minute: .... 5 minutes: ....

Apgar Scoring:

Sl No.	*Signs*	*0*	*Neonate's Score*	*1*	*Neonates Score*	*2*	*Neonates' Score*
1.	Respiratory effort	Absent		Slow, irregular, weak, cry		Strong cry	
2.	Heart rate	Absent		Slow < 100		Over 100	
3.	Muscle tone	Limb		Some flexion of limbs		Active movement	
4.	Reflex response to flecking of foot	Absent		Facial grimace		Cry	
5.	Color	Blue-pale		Body is pink Limbs are blue		Completely pink	

Birth Injury: Yes/No: If 'Yes' specify: ....

c. Physical Examination: General Appearance and Posture

i. Anthropometric Measurements:

Birth weight: .... kg

Head to heel length: .... cm

Head circumference: .... cm

Chest circumference: .... cm

ii. Vital Signs:

Temperature (Auxiliary): ....

Heart Rate (Apical): ....

Respiration: ....

iii. Skin:

Color: Normal/Pale/Cyanosed/Jaundice: ....

Lanugo: Present/Absent: ....

Vernix caseosa: ....

Rash: Present/Absent: ....

Milia: Present/Absent: ....

Mongolian Spots: Present/Absent: ....

Texture: Normal/Dry/Edematous: ....

Erythema Toxicum: Present/Absent: ....

iv. Head:

Size: ....

Fontanelle: ....

Sutures: ....

Caput succedaneum: ....

Cephalohematoma: ....

Any Other: ....

v. Eyes:

Blink reflex: ....

Conjunctiva: ....

Cornea: ....

Discharge: ....

Any other: ....

vi. Ears:

Position: ....

Recoiling of pinna: ....

vii. Nose:

Nasal flaring: ....

Discharge: ....

Any other: ....

viii. Mouth and Throat:

Color of lips: ....

Color of tongue: ....

Palate: ....

Cry: ....

ix. Neck: ....

x. Chest:

Breath sounds: ....

Apnea: ....

Stridor: ....

xi. Breast: ....

xii. Abdomen:

Umbilical stump: ....

Bowel sounds: ....

Any other abnormality: ....

xiii. Spine: ....

xiv. Extremities:

Palmar creases: ....

Plantar creases: ....

Deformity: ....

xv. Genitourinary:

Female: Vaginal discharge: ....

Male: Normal/Hypospadias/Hydrocele: ....

Testis: Descended/Undescended: ....

Ambiguous Genitalia: Yes/No: ....

xvi. Rectum:

Anal patency: ....

Anal excoriation: ....

xvii. Neurological Reflexes:

Moro reflexes: ....

Stepping or dancing reflexes: ....

Glabellar reflexes: ....

Tonic neck reflexes: ....

Grasping reflexes: ....

Babinski reflexes: ....

Rooting: ....

Sucking: ....

Swallowing: ....

Gag: ....

Blinking: ....

Cough and sneeze: ....

Yawn: ....

Other neuromuscular manifestation: Absent/Hypotonic/Hypertonic/Opisthotonos/Jitteriness:

....

Seizures: ....

d. Investigation:

Date	*Type of Investigation*	*Newborn's Value*	*Normal Value*	*Interpretation*
1.				
2.				
3.				
4.				
5.				
6.				

e. Medications:

Date	*Name/Dosage/Frequency/ Route*	*Action*	*Side Effect*	*Nursing Responsibility*

NURSING CARE PLAN

Assessment	*Nursing Diagnosis*	*Goals*	*Nursing Intervention*	*Rationale*	*Nursing Implementation*	*Evaluation*

NURSING CARE PLAN

Assessment	*Nursing Diagnosis*	*Goals*	*Nursing Intervention*	*Rationale*	*Nursing Implementation*	*Evaluation*

NURSING CARE PLAN

Assessment	*Nursing Diagnosis*	*Goals*	*Nursing Intervention*	*Rationale*	*Nursing Implementation*	*Evaluation*

ASSESSMENT AND CARE OF THE NEWBORN (2)

1. Profile of the Newborn:

   Name: ....

   Name of the Hospital: ....

   Inpatient (IP) Number (No): .... Ward: ....

   Mother's Name: ....

   Father's Name: ....

   Address: ....

   Date of Birth: .... Sex: Male/Female: ....

   Birth Order: ....

   Apgar Score:

   1 minute: .... 5 minutes: ....

   Religion: ....

   Educational Status:

   Mother: .... Father: ....

   Occupation:

   Father: .... Mother: ....

   Total income of the family: ....

2. Birth History:

   a. Antenatal history:

      Age of mother: ....

      Type of marriage:

      Consanguineous: .... Nonconsanguineous: ....

      Degree of consanguinity: ....

      Antenatal checkups:

      Regular: .... Irregular: ....

      Tetanus toxoid:

      Yes/No: .... No. of doses: ....

      Any exposure to drug/radiation: ....

      If Yes: Specify: ....

      Any illness during pregnancy: ....

b. Intranatal History:

Date and time of delivery: ....

Place of delivery: ....

Delivery conducted by: ....

Mode of delivery: ....

Gestational age (in weeks): ....

Birth weight: .... kg

Cried at birth: Yes/No: ....

Apgar score: 1 minute: .... 5 minutes: ....

Apgar Scoring:

Sl No.	*Signs*	*0*	*Neonate's Score*	*1*	*Neonates Score*	*2*	*Neonates' Score*
1.	Respiratory effort	Absent		Slow, irregular, weak, cry		Strong cry	
2.	Heart rate	Absent		Slow < 100		Over 100	
3.	Muscle tone	Limb		Some flexion of limbs		Active movement	
4.	Reflex response to flecking of foot	Absent		Facial grimace		Cry	
5.	Color	Blue-pale		Body is pink Limbs are blue		Completely pink	

Birth Injury: Yes/No: If 'Yes' specify: ....

c. Physical Examination: General Appearance and Posture

i. Anthropometric Measurements:

Birth weight: .... kg

Head to heel length: .... cm

Head circumference: .... cm

Chest circumference: .... cm

ii. Vital Signs:

Temperature (Auxiliary): ....

Heart Rate (Apical): ....

Respiration: ....

iii. Skin:

Color: Normal/Pale/Cyanosed/Jaundice: ....

Lanugo: Present/Absent: ....

Vernix caseosa: ....

Rash: Present/Absent: ....

Milia: Present/Absent: ....

Mongolian Spots: Present/Absent: ....

Texture: Normal/Dry/Edematous: ....

Erythema Toxicum: Present/Absent: ....

iv. Head:

Size: ....

Fontanelle: ....

Sutures: ....

Caput succedaneum: ....

Cephalohematoma: ....

Any Other: ....

v. Eyes:

Blink reflex: ....

Conjunctiva: ....

Cornea: ....

Discharge: ....

Any other: ....

vi. Ears:

Position: ....

Recoiling of pinna: ....

vii. Nose:

Nasal flaring: ....

Discharge: ....

Any other: ....

viii. Mouth and Throat:

Color of lips: ....

Color of tongue: ....

Palate: ....

Cry: ....

ix. Neck: ....

x. Chest:

Breath sounds: ....

Apnea: ....

Stridor: ....

xi. Breast: ....

xii. Abdomen:

Umbilical stump: ....

Bowel sounds: ....

Any other abnormality: ....

xiii. Spine: ....

xiv. Extremities:

Palmar creases: ....

Plantar creases: ....

Deformity: ....

xv. Genitourinary:

Female: Vaginal discharge: ....

Male: Normal/Hypospadias/Hydrocele: ....

Testis: Descended/Undescended: ....

Ambiguous Genitalia: Yes/No: ....

xvi. Rectum:

Anal patency: ....

Anal excoriation: ....

xvii. Neurological Reflexes:

Moro reflexes: ....

Stepping or dancing reflexes: ....

Glabellar reflexes: ....

Tonic neck reflexes: ....

Grasping reflexes: ....

Babinski reflexes: ....

Rooting: ....

Sucking: ....

Swallowing: ....

Gag: ....

Blinking: ....

Cough and sneeze: ....

Yawn: ....

Other neuromuscular manifestation: Absent/Hypotonic/Hypertonic/Opisthotonos/Jitteriness:

....

Seizures: ....

d. Investigation:

Date	*Type of Investigation*	*Newborn's Value*	*Normal Value*	*Interpretation*
1.				
2.				
3.				
4.				
5.				
6.				

e. Medications:

Date	*Name/Dosage/Frequency/ Route*	*Action*	*Side Effect*	*Nursing Responsibility*

NURSING CARE PLAN

Assessment	*Nursing Diagnosis*	*Goals*	*Nursing Intervention*	*Rationale*	*Nursing Implementation*	*Evaluation*

NURSING CARE PLAN

Assessment	*Nursing Diagnosis*	*Goals*	*Nursing Intervention*	*Rationale*	*Nursing Implementation*	*Evaluation*

NURSING CARE PLAN

Assessment	*Nursing Diagnosis*	*Goals*	*Nursing Intervention*	*Rationale*	*Nursing Implementation*	*Evaluation*

ASSESSMENT AND CARE OF THE NEWBORN (3)

1. Profile of the Newborn:

   Name: ....

   Name of the Hospital: ....

   Inpatient (IP) Number (No): .... Ward: ....

   Mother's Name: ....

   Father's Name: ....

   Address: ....

   Date of Birth: .... Sex: Male/Female: ....

   Birth Order: ....

   Apgar Score:

   1 minute: .... 5 minutes: ....

   Religion: ....

   Educational Status:

   Mother: .... Father: ....

   Occupation:

   Father: .... Mother: ....

   Total income of the family: ....

2. Birth History:

   a. Antenatal history:

      Age of mother: ....

      Type of marriage:

      Consanguineous: .... Nonconsanguineous: ....

      Degree of consanguinity: ....

      Antenatal checkups:

      Regular: .... Irregular: ....

      Tetanus toxoid:

      Yes/No: .... No. of doses: ....

      Any exposure to drug/radiation: ....

      If Yes: Specify: ....

      Any illness during pregnancy: ....

b. Intranatal History:

Date and time of delivery: ....

Place of delivery: ....

Delivery conducted by: ....

Mode of delivery: ....

Gestational age (in weeks): ....

Birth weight: .... kg

Cried at birth: Yes/No: ....

Apgar score: 1 minute: .... 5 minutes: ....

Apgar Scoring:

Sl No.	*Signs*	*0*	*Neonate's Score*	*1*	*Neonates Score*	*2*	*Neonates' Score*
1.	Respiratory effort	Absent		Slow, irregular, weak, cry		Strong cry	
2.	Heart rate	Absent		Slow < 100		Over 100	
3.	Muscle tone	Limb		Some flexion of limbs		Active movement	
4.	Reflex response to flecking of foot	Absent		Facial grimace		Cry	
5.	Color	Blue-pale		Body is pink Limbs are blue		Completely pink	

Birth Injury: Yes/No: If 'Yes' specify: ....

c. Physical Examination: General Appearance and Posture

i. Anthropometric Measurements:

Birth weight: .... kg

Head to heel length: .... cm

Head circumference: .... cm

Chest circumference: .... cm

ii. Vital Signs:

Temperature (Auxiliary): ....

Heart Rate (Apical): ....

Respiration: ....

iii. Skin:

Color: Normal/Pale/Cyanosed/Jaundice: ....

Lanugo: Present/Absent: ....

Vernix caseosa: ....

Rash: Present/Absent: ....

Milia: Present/Absent: ....

Mongolian Spots: Present/Absent: ....

Texture: Normal/Dry/Edematous: ....

Erythema Toxicum: Present/Absent: ....

iv. Head:

Size: ....

Fontanelle: ....

Sutures: ....

Caput succedaneum: ....

Cephalohematoma: ....

Any Other: ....

v. Eyes:

Blink reflex: ....

Conjunctiva: ....

Cornea: ....

Discharge: ....

Any other: ....

vi. Ears:

Position: ....

Recoiling of pinna: ....

vii. Nose:

Nasal flaring: ....

Discharge: ....

Any other: ....

viii. Mouth and Throat:

Color of lips: ....

Color of tongue: ....

Palate: ....

Cry: ....

ix. Neck: ....

x. Chest:

Breath sounds: ....

Apnea: ....

Stridor: ....

xi. Breast: ....

xii. Abdomen:

Umbilical stump: ....

Bowel sounds: ....

Any other abnormality: ....

xiii. Spine: ....

xiv. Extremities:

Palmar creases: ....

Plantar creases: ....

Deformity: ....

xv. Genitourinary:

Female: Vaginal discharge: ....

Male: Normal/Hypospadias/Hydrocele: ....

Testis: Descended/Undescended: ....

Ambiguous Genitalia: Yes/No: ....

xvi. Rectum:

Anal patency: ....

Anal excoriation: ....

xvii. Neurological Reflexes:

Moro reflexes: ....

Stepping or dancing reflexes: ....

Glabellar reflexes: ....

Tonic neck reflexes: ....

Grasping reflexes: ....

Babinski reflexes: ....

Rooting: ....

Sucking: ....

Swallowing: ....

Gag: ....

Blinking: ....

Cough and sneeze: ....

Yawn: ....

Other neuromuscular manifestation: Absent/Hypotonic/Hypertonic/Opisthotonos/Jitteriness: ....

Seizures: ....

d. Investigation:

Date	*Type of Investigation*	*Newborn's Value*	*Normal Value*	*Interpretation*
1.				
2.				
3.				
4.				
5.				
6.				

e. Medications:

Date	*Name/Dosage/Frequency/ Route*	*Action*	*Side Effect*	*Nursing Responsibility*

NURSING CARE PLAN

Assessment	*Nursing Diagnosis*	*Goals*	*Nursing Intervention*	*Rationale*	*Nursing Implementation*	*Evaluation*

NURSING CARE PLAN

Assessment	*Nursing Diagnosis*	*Goals*	*Nursing Intervention*	*Rationale*	*Nursing Implementation*	*Evaluation*

NURSING CARE PLAN

Assessment	*Nursing Diagnosis*	*Goals*	*Nursing Intervention*	*Rationale*	*Nursing Implementation*	*Evaluation*

ASSESSMENT AND CARE OF THE NEWBORN (4)

1. Profile of the Newborn:

   Name: ....

   Name of the Hospital: ....

   Inpatient (IP) Number (No): .... Ward: ....

   Mother's Name: ....

   Father's Name: ....

   Address: ....

   Date of Birth: .... Sex: Male/Female: ....

   Birth Order: ....

   Apgar Score:

   1 minute: .... 5 minutes: ....

   Religion: ....

   Educational Status:

   Mother: .... Father: ....

   Occupation:

   Father: .... Mother: ....

   Total income of the family: ....

2. Birth History:

   a. Antenatal history:

      Age of mother: ....

      Type of marriage:

      Consanguineous: .... Nonconsanguineous: ....

      Degree of consanguinity: ....

      Antenatal checkups:

      Regular: .... Irregular: ....

      Tetanus toxoid:

      Yes/No: .... No. of doses: ....

      Any exposure to drug/radiation: ....

      If Yes: Specify: ....

      Any illness during pregnancy: ....

b. Intranatal History:

Date and time of delivery: ....

Place of delivery: ....

Delivery conducted by: ....

Mode of delivery: ....

Gestational age (in weeks): ....

Birth weight: .... kg

Cried at birth: Yes/No: ....

Apgar score: 1 minute: .... 5 minutes: ....

Apgar Scoring:

Sl No.	*Signs*	*0*	*Neonate's Score*	*1*	*Neonates Score*	*2*	*Neonates' Score*
1.	Respiratory effort	Absent		Slow, irregular, weak, cry		Strong cry	
2.	Heart rate	Absent		Slow < 100		Over 100	
3.	Muscle tone	Limb		Some flexion of limbs		Active movement	
4.	Reflex response to flecking of foot	Absent		Facial grimace		Cry	
5.	Color	Blue-pale		Body is pink Limbs are blue		Completely pink	

Birth Injury: Yes/No: If 'Yes' specify: ....

c. Physical Examination: General Appearance and Posture

i. Anthropometric Measurements:

Birth weight: .... kg

Head to heel length: .... cm

Head circumference: .... cm

Chest circumference: .... cm

ii. Vital Signs:

Temperature (Auxiliary): ....

Heart Rate (Apical): ....

Respiration: ....

iii. Skin:

Color: Normal/Pale/Cyanosed/Jaundice: ....

Lanugo: Present/Absent: ....

Vernix caseosa: ....

Rash: Present/Absent: ....

Milia: Present/Absent: ....

Mongolian Spots: Present/Absent: ....

Texture: Normal/Dry/Edematous: ....

Erythema Toxicum: Present/Absent: ....

iv. Head:

Size: ....

Fontanelle: ....

Sutures: ....

Caput succedaneum: ....

Cephalohematoma: ....

Any Other: ....

v. Eyes:

Blink reflex: ....

Conjunctiva: ....

Cornea: ....

Discharge: ....

Any other: ....

vi. Ears:

Position: ....

Recoiling of pinna: ....

vii. Nose:

Nasal flaring: ....

Discharge: ....

Any other: ....

viii. Mouth and Throat:

Color of lips: ....

Color of tongue: ....

Palate: ....

Cry: ....

ix. Neck: ....

x. Chest:

Breath sounds: ....

Apnea: ....

Stridor: ....

xi. Breast: ....

xii. Abdomen:

Umbilical stump: ....

Bowel sounds: ....

Any other abnormality: ....

xiii. Spine: ....

xiv. Extremities:

Palmar creases: ....

Plantar creases: ....

Deformity: ....

xv. Genitourinary:

Female: Vaginal discharge: ....

Male: Normal/Hypospadias/Hydrocele: ....

Testis: Descended/Undescended: ....

Ambiguous Genitalia: Yes/No: ....

xvi. Rectum:

Anal patency: ....

Anal excoriation: ....

xvii. Neurological Reflexes:

Moro reflexes: ....

Stepping or dancing reflexes: ....

Glabellar reflexes: ....

Tonic neck reflexes: ....

Grasping reflexes: ....

Babinski reflexes: ....

Rooting: ....

Sucking: ....

Swallowing: ....

Gag: ....

Blinking: ....

Cough and sneeze: ....

Yawn: ....

Other neuromuscular manifestation: Absent/Hypotonic/Hypertonic/Opisthotonos/Jitteriness: ....

Seizures: ....

d. Investigation:

Date	*Type of Investigation*	*Newborn's Value*	*Normal Value*	*Interpretation*
1.				
2.				
3.				
4.				
5.				
6.				

e. Medications:

Date	*Name/Dosage/Frequency/ Route*	*Action*	*Side Effect*	*Nursing Responsibility*

NURSING CARE PLAN

Assessment	*Nursing Diagnosis*	*Goals*	*Nursing Intervention*	*Rationale*	*Nursing Implementation*	*Evaluation*

NURSING CARE PLAN

Assessment	*Nursing Diagnosis*	*Goals*	*Nursing Intervention*	*Rationale*	*Nursing Implementation*	*Evaluation*

NURSING CARE PLAN

Assessment	*Nursing Diagnosis*	*Goals*	*Nursing Intervention*	*Rationale*	*Nursing Implementation*	*Evaluation*

ASSESSMENT AND CARE OF THE NEWBORN (5)

1. Profile of the Newborn:

   Name: ....

   Name of the Hospital: ....

   Inpatient (IP) Number (No): .... Ward: ....

   Mother's Name: ....

   Father's Name: ....

   Address: ....

   Date of Birth: .... Sex: Male/Female: ....

   Birth Order: ....

   Apgar Score:

   1 minute: .... 5 minutes: ....

   Religion: ....

   Educational Status:

   Mother: .... Father: ....

   Occupation:

   Father: .... Mother: ....

   Total income of the family: ....

2. Birth History:

   a. Antenatal history:

      Age of mother: ....

      Type of marriage:

      Consanguineous: .... Nonconsanguineous: ....

      Degree of consanguinity: ....

      Antenatal checkups:

      Regular: .... Irregular: ....

      Tetanus toxoid:

      Yes/No: .... No. of doses: ....

      Any exposure to drug/radiation: ....

      If Yes: Specify: ....

      Any illness during pregnancy: ....

b. Intranatal History:

Date and time of delivery: ....

Place of delivery: ....

Delivery conducted by: ....

Mode of delivery: ....

Gestational age (in weeks): ....

Birth weight: .... kg

Cried at birth: Yes/No: ....

Apgar score: 1 minute: .... 5 minutes: ....

Apgar Scoring:

Sl No.	*Signs*	*0*	*Neonate's Score*	*1*	*Neonates Score*	*2*	*Neonates' Score*
1.	Respiratory effort	Absent		Slow, irregular, weak, cry		Strong cry	
2.	Heart rate	Absent		Slow < 100		Over 100	
3.	Muscle tone	Limb		Some flexion of limbs		Active movement	
4.	Reflex response to flecking of foot	Absent		Facial grimace		Cry	
5.	Color	Blue-pale		Body is pink Limbs are blue		Completely pink	

Birth Injury: Yes/No: If 'Yes' specify: ....

c. Physical Examination: General Appearance and Posture

i. Anthropometric Measurements:

Birth weight: .... kg

Head to heel length: .... cm

Head circumference: .... cm

Chest circumference: .... cm

ii. Vital Signs:

Temperature (Auxiliary): ....

Heart Rate (Apical): ....

Respiration: ....

iii. Skin:

Color: Normal/Pale/Cyanosed/Jaundice: ....

Lanugo: Present/Absent: ....

Vernix caseosa: ....

Rash: Present/Absent: ....

Milia: Present/Absent: ....

Mongolian Spots: Present/Absent: ....

Texture: Normal/Dry/Edematous: ....

Erythema Toxicum: Present/Absent: ....

iv. Head:

Size: ....

Fontanelle: ....

Sutures: ....

Caput succedaneum: ....

Cephalohematoma: ....

Any Other: ....

v. Eyes:

Blink reflex: ....

Conjunctiva: ....

Cornea: ....

Discharge: ....

Any other: ....

vi. Ears:

Position: ....

Recoiling of pinna: ....

vii. Nose:

Nasal flaring: ....

Discharge: ....

Any other: ....

viii. Mouth and Throat:

Color of lips: ....

Color of tongue: ....

Palate: ....

Cry: ....

ix. Neck: ....

x. Chest:

Breath sounds: ....

Apnea: ....

Stridor: ....

xi. Breast: ....

xii. Abdomen:

Umbilical stump: ....

Bowel sounds: ....

Any other abnormality: ....

xiii. Spine: ....

xiv. Extremities:

Palmar creases: ....

Plantar creases: ....

Deformity: ....

xv. Genitourinary:

Female: Vaginal discharge: ....

Male: Normal/Hypospadias/Hydrocele: ....

Testis: Descended/Undescended: ....

Ambiguous Genitalia: Yes/No: ....

xvi. Rectum:

Anal patency: ....

Anal excoriation: ....

xvii. Neurological Reflexes:

Moro reflexes: ....

Stepping or dancing reflexes: ....

Glabellar reflexes: ....

Tonic neck reflexes: ....

Grasping reflexes: ....

Babinski reflexes: ....

Rooting: ....

Sucking: ....

Swallowing: ....

Gag: ....

Blinking: ....

Cough and sneeze: ....

Yawn: ....

Other neuromuscular manifestation: Absent/Hypotonic/Hypertonic/Opisthotonos/Jitteriness: ....

Seizures: ....

d. Investigation:

Date	*Type of Investigation*	*Newborn's Value*	*Normal Value*	*Interpretation*
1.				
2.				
3.				
4.				
5.				
6.				

e. Medications:

Date	*Name/Dosage/Frequency/ Route*	*Action*	*Side Effect*	*Nursing Responsibility*

NURSING CARE PLAN

Assessment	*Nursing Diagnosis*	*Goals*	*Nursing Intervention*	*Rationale*	*Nursing Implementation*	*Evaluation*

NURSING CARE PLAN

Assessment	*Nursing Diagnosis*	*Goals*	*Nursing Intervention*	*Rationale*	*Nursing Implementation*	*Evaluation*

NURSING CARE PLAN

Assessment	Nursing Diagnosis	Goals	Nursing Intervention	Rationale	Nursing Implementation	Evaluation

CHAPTER 8

Cesarean Section Witnessed/Assisted

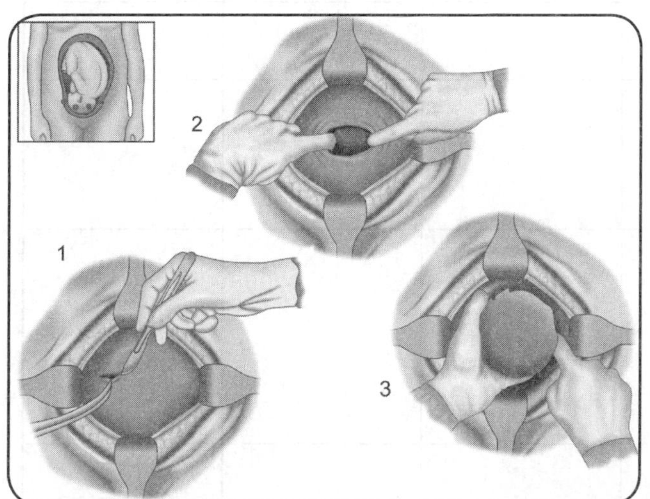

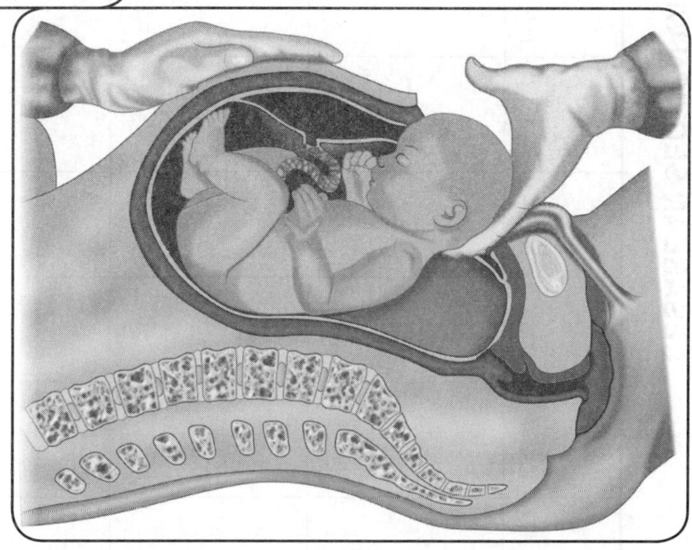

CESAREAN SECTION WITNESSED/ASSISTED

Sl No.	*IP No.*	*Name of the Mother*	*Age*	*Obstetrical Score*	*LMP*	*EDD*	*Gestational Age*	*Indication*	*Procedure Performed*	*Conditions of the Mother*	*Condition of the Baby*			*Performed by*
											Weight (kg)	*Sex*	*Apgar Score*	
1.														
2.														
3.														
4.														
5.														

Signature of the Students

Signature of the Supervisor

CHAPTER 9

Abnormal Deliveries Witnessed/Assisted

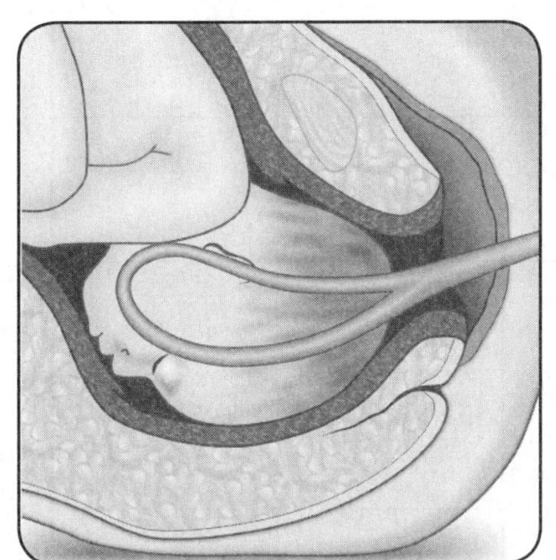

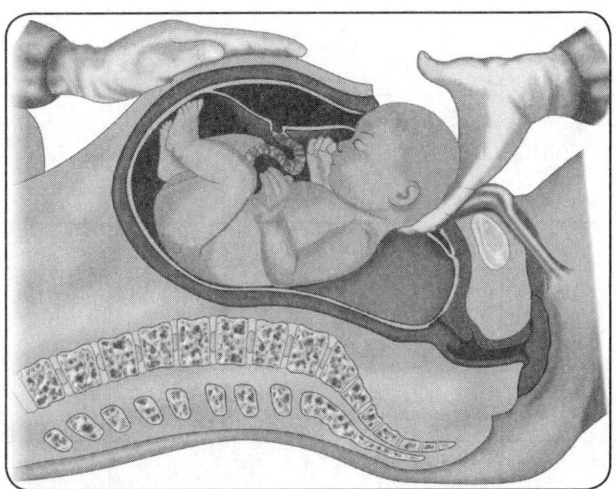

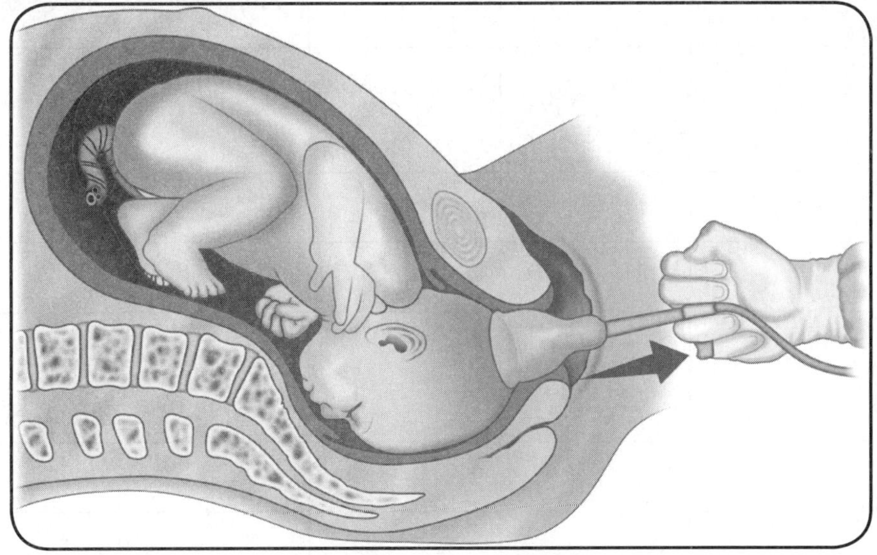

ABNORMAL DELIVERIES WITNESSED/ASSISTED
(Forceps, Ventouse, Breech, Twins, Occipitoposterior, Face Presentation)

Sl No.	*IP No.*	*Name of the Mother*	*Age*	*Obstetrical Score*	*LMP*	*EDD*	*Gestational Age*	*Indication*	*Procedures Performed*	*Conditions of the Mother*	*Condition of the Baby*			*Performed by*
											Weight (kg)	*Sex*	*Apgar Score*	
1.														
2.														
3.														
4.														
5.														

Signature of the Supervisor

CHAPTER 10

Assisted for Neonatal Resuscitation

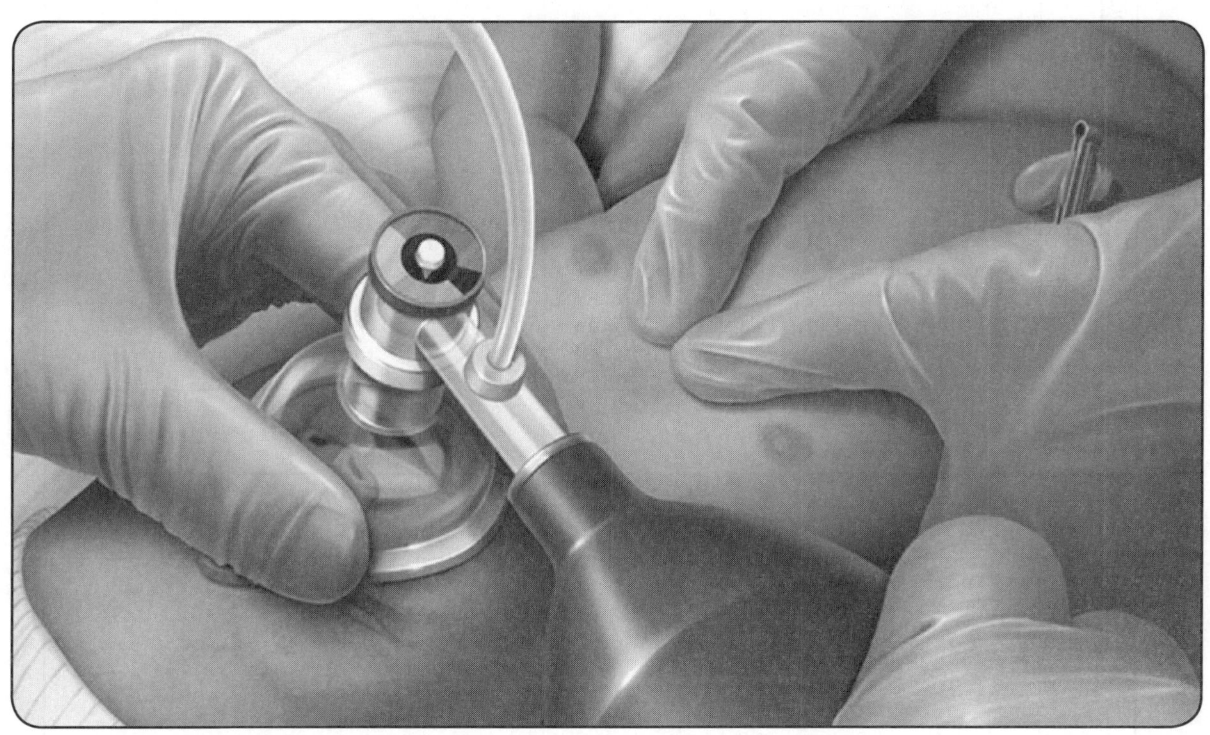

ASSISTED FOR NEONATAL RESUSCITATION (1)

Sl No.	IP No.	Name of the Baby	Date of Birth	Nature of the Delivery	Apgar Score		Resuscitation		
					1 min	5 min	Indications	Measures	Condition after Procedure
1.									
2.									

Signature of the Supervisor

ASSISTED FOR NEONATAL RESUSCITATION (2)

Sl No.	*IP No.*	*Name of the Baby*	*Date of Birth*	*Nature of the Delivery*	*Apgar Score*		*Resuscitation*		
					1 min	*5 min*	*Indications*	*Measures*	*Condition after Procedure*
1.									
2.									

Signature of the Supervisor

CHAPTER 11

Assisted for Dilation and Evacuation Procedure

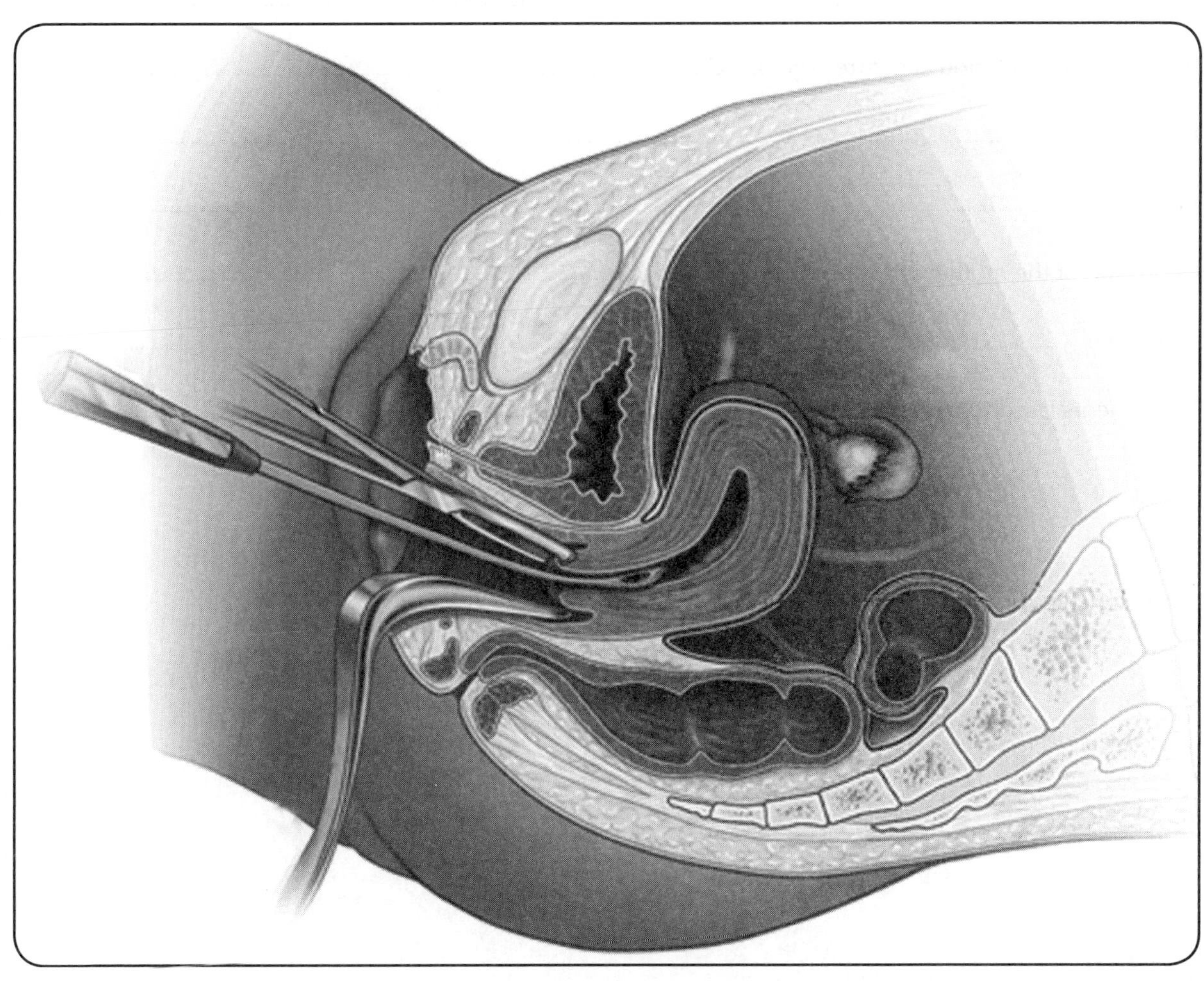

ASSISTED IN DILATION AND EVACUATION (1)

Name of the Mother: .... Age: .... IP No: ....

Religion: .... Date of Admission: ....

Educational Status: .... Date of Procedure Done: ....

Occupation: .... LMP: ....

Obstetrical score: .... EDD: ....

Blood Group: .... Gestational age: ....

Indication for dialation and curettage (D&C): ....

Prepreparation: ....

Procedures: ....

Condition of the mother after the procedure: ....

Aftercare: ....

Instruments Used (draw instruments with purpose): ....

Signature of the Student

Signature of the Supervisor

ASSISTED IN DILATION AND EVACUATION (2)

Name of the Mother: .... Age: .... IP No: ....

Religion: .... Date of Admission: ....

Educational Status: .... Date of Procedure Done: ....

Occupation: .... LMP: ....

Obstetrical score: .... EDD: ....

Blood Group: .... Gestational age: ....

Indication for dialation and curettage (D&C): ....

Prepreparation: ....

Procedures: ....

Condition of the mother after the procedure: ....

Aftercare: ....

Instruments Used (draw instruments with purpose): ....

Signature of the Student

Signature of the Supervisor

INSTRUMENTS USED (DRAW INSTRUMENTS WITH PURPOSE)

CHAPTER 12

Assisted for Female Sterilization (Tubectomy)

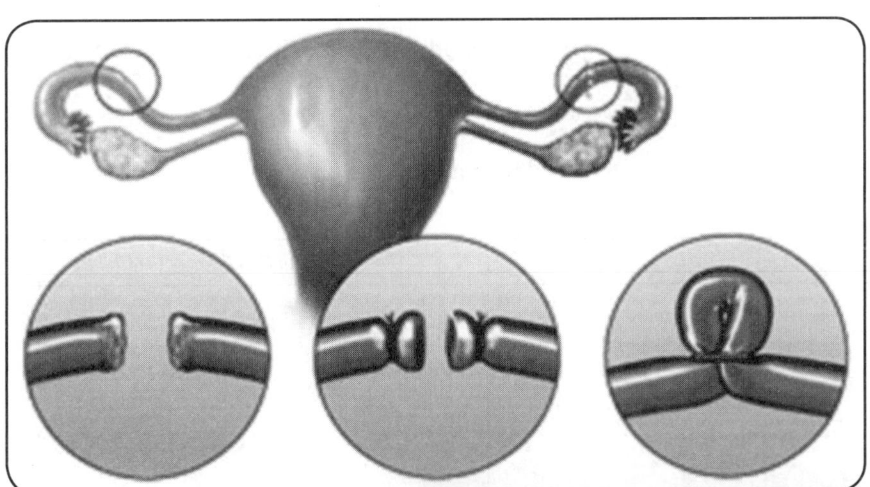

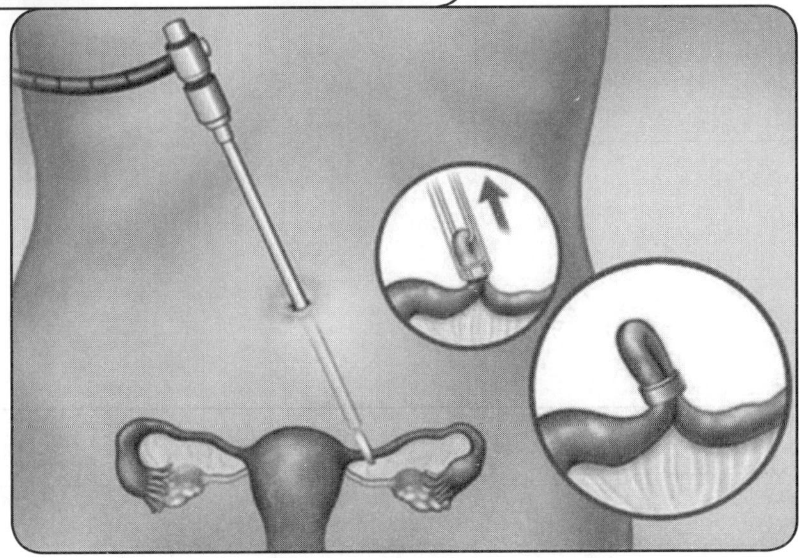

ASSISTED FOR FEMALE STERILIZATION (TUBECTOMY) (1)

Name of the Mother: .... Age: ....

Date of Admission: .... IP No.: ....

Educational Status: .... Wife: ....

Husband: ....

Occupation: .... Wife: ....

Husband: ....

Religion: .... Wife: ....

Husband: ....

No. of Living Children	*Age*	*Sex*	*Health Condition of the Children*

Preparation of the mother: ....

....

....

Physical preparation: ....

Premedications: ....

Consent form: ....

Psychological preparation: ....

Time of operation performed: ....

Procedure or method: ....

Performed by: ....

Conditions of the procedure are performed: ....

Conditions of the mother: ....

Aftercare and advice to the mother: ....

Signature of the Supervisor

ASSISTED FOR FEMALE STERILIZATION (TUBECTOMY) (2)

Name of the Mother: .... Age: ....

Date of Admission: .... IP No.: ....

Educational Status: .... Wife: ....

Husband: ....

Occupation: .... Wife: ....

Husband: ....

Religion: .... Wife: ....

Husband: ....

No. of Living Children	*Age*	*Sex*	*Health Condition of the Children*

Preparation of the mother: ....

....

....

Physical preparation: ....

Premedications: ....

Consent form: ....

Psychological preparation: ....

Time of operation performed: ....

Procedure or method: ....

Performed by: ....

Conditions of the procedure are performed: ....

Conditions of the mother: ....

Aftercare and advice to the mother: ....

Signature of the Supervisor

ASSISTED FOR FEMALE STERILIZATION (TUBECTOMY) (3)

Name of the Mother: .... Age: ....

Date of Admission: .... IP No.: ....

Educational Status: .... Wife: ....

Husband: ....

Occupation: .... Wife: ....

Husband: ....

Religion: .... Wife: ....

Husband: ....

No. of Living Children	*Age*	*Sex*	*Health Condition of the Children*

Preparation of the mother: ....

....

....

Physical preparation: ....

Premedications: ....

Consent form: ....

Psychological preparation: ....

Time of operation performed: ....

Procedure or method: ....

Performed by: ....

Conditions of the procedure are performed: ....

Conditions of the mother: ....

Aftercare and advice to the mother: ....

Signature of the Supervisor

ASSISTED FOR FEMALE STERILIZATION (TUBECTOMY) (4)

Name of the Mother: .... Age: ....

Date of Admission: .... IP No.: ....

Educational Status: .... Wife: ....

Husband: ....

Occupation: .... Wife: ....

Husband: ....

Religion: .... Wife: ....

Husband: ....

No. of Living Children	*Age*	*Sex*	*Health Condition of the Children*

Preparation of the mother: ....

....

....

Physical preparation: ....

Premedications: ....

Consent form: ....

Psychological preparation: ....

Time of operation performed: ....

Procedure or method: ....

Performed by: ....

Conditions of the procedure are performed: ....

Conditions of the mother: ....

Aftercare and advice to the mother: ....

Signature of the Supervisor

CHAPTER 13

Assisted for Male Sterilization (Vasectomy)

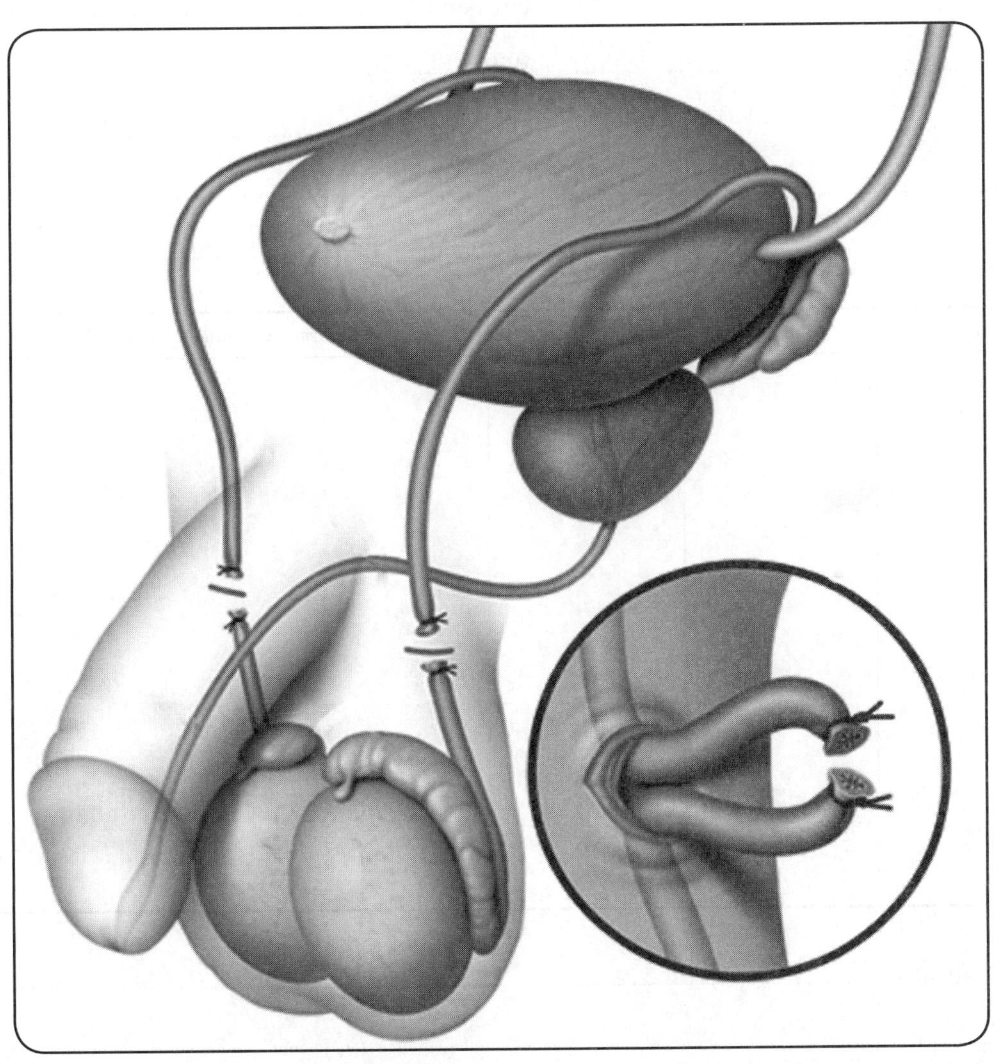

ASSISTED FOR MALE STERILIZATION (VASECTOMY)

Name of the Patient: .... Date of Admission: ....

Age: .... IP No.: ....

Educational Status: .... Wife: ....

Husband: ....

Religion: .... Wife: ....

Husband: ....

Occupation: .... Wife: ....

Husband: ....

No. of Living Children	*Age*	*Sex*	*Health Condition of the Children*

Preparation of the patient: ....

....

....

Physical preparation: ....

Premedications: ....

Consent form: ....

Psychological preparation: ....

Time of operation performed: ....

Procedure or method: ....

Performed by: ....

Condition of the procedure is performed: ....

Conditions of the patient: ....

Aftercare and advice to the mother: ....

Signature of the Supervisor

CHAPTER 14

Motivation for Planned Parenthood

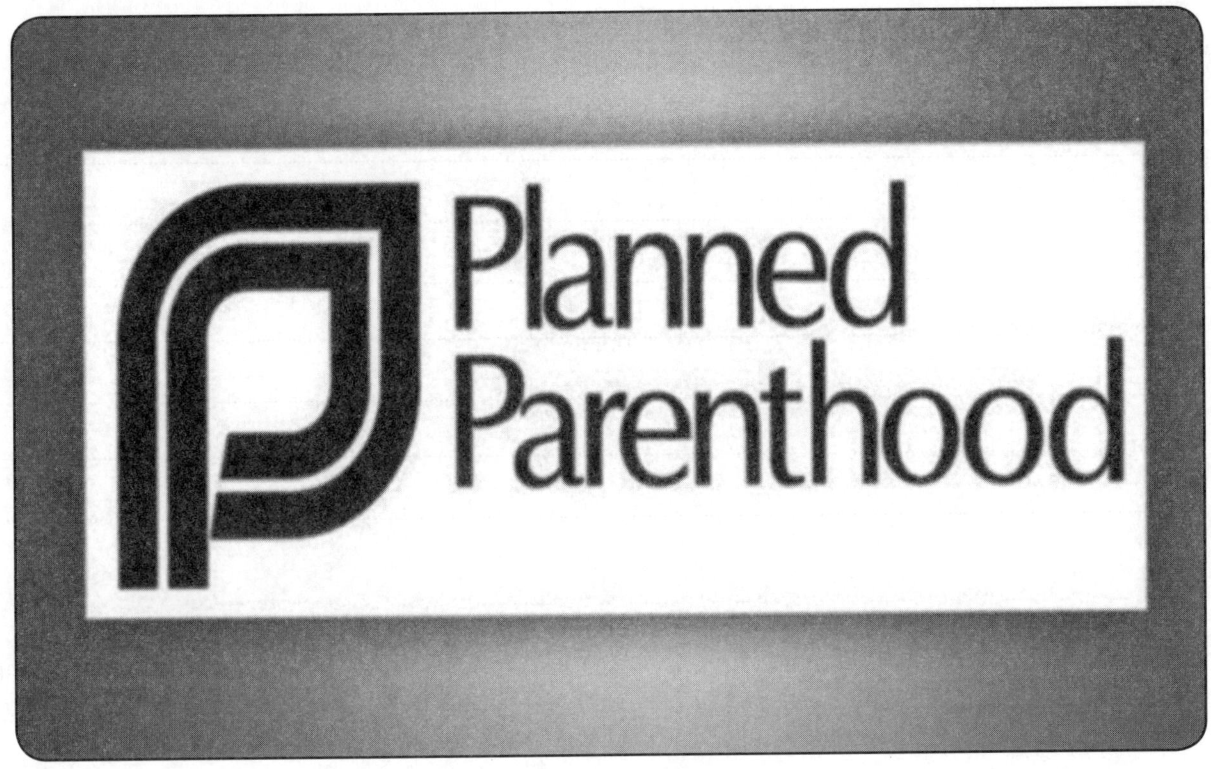

MOTIVATION FOR PLANNED PARENTHOOD (1)

Name of the Mother: .... Name of the Father: ....

Age: .... Age: ....

Educational Status: .... Educational Status: ....

Occupation: .... Occupation: ....

Marital status: ....

Advice to the parents: ....

....

....

....

Audiovisual aids used: ....

....

Remarks: ....

....

Signature of the Student

Signature of the Supervisor

MOTIVATION FOR PLANNED PARENTHOOD (2)

Name of the Mother: .... Name of the Father: ....

Age: .... Age: ....

Educational Status: .... Educational Status: ....

Occupation: .... Occupation: ....

Marital status: ....

Advice to the parents: ....

....

....

....

Audiovisual aids used: ....

....

Remarks: ....

....

Signature of the Student Signature of the Supervisor

CHAPTER 15

Assisted for IUCD Insertions

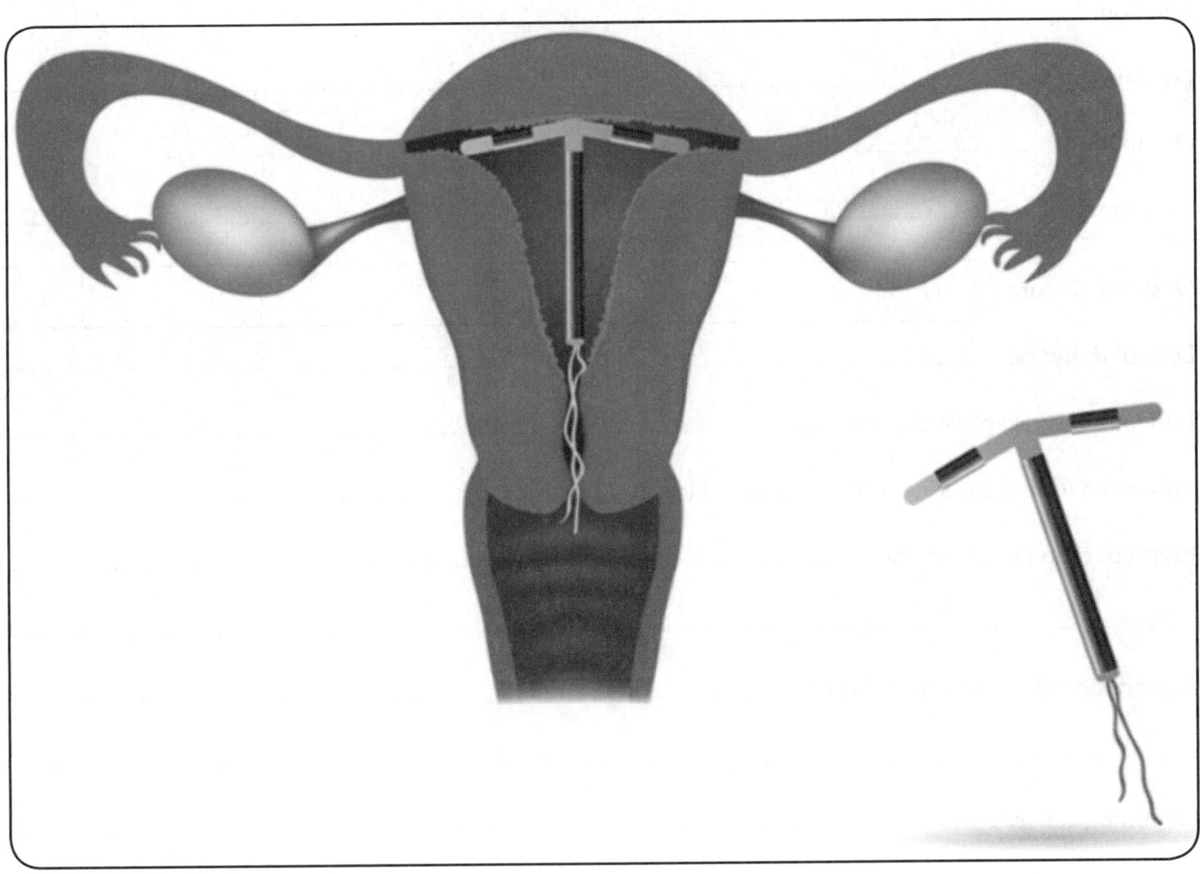

ASSISTED FOR IUCD INSERTIONS (1)

Basic Profile of the Mother:

Name of the Mother: ....

Age: .... years

Religion: ....

Educational Status: ....

Occupation: ....

Register No.: ....

Obstetrical score:

G		P		L		A		S		D	

Date of delivery: ....

Previous contraceptive history: ....

Indication for intrauterine contraceptive device (IUCD) insertion: ....

Prepreparation of the mother: ....

....

Explanation about the procedure: ....

....

Obtaining consent form: ....

Preparation of the articles: ....

....

....

Specific instruction to the mother: ....

....

....

Types of IUCD used: ....

Procedure of IUCD insertion: ....

....

....

....

....

Aftercare and advice to the mother: ....

....

Remarks: ....

Signature of the Student Signature of the Supervisor

Instruction: ....

....

ASSISTED FOR IUCD INSERTIONS (2)

Basic Profile of the Mother:

Name of the Mother: ....

Age: .... years

Religion: ....

Educational Status: ....

Occupation: ....

Register No.: ....

Obstetrical score:

G		P		L		A		S		D	

Date of delivery: ....

Previous contraceptive history: ....

Indication for intrauterine contraceptive device (IUCD) insertion: ....

Prepreparation of the mother: ....

....

Explanation about the procedure: ....

....

Obtaining consent form: ....

Preparation of the articles: ....

....

....

Specific instruction to the mother: ....

....

....

Types of IUCD used: ....

Procedure of IUCD insertion: ....

....

....

....

....

Aftercare and advice to the mother: ....

....

Remarks: ....

Signature of the Student | Signature of the Supervisor

Instruction: ....

....

ASSISTED FOR IUCD INSERTIONS (3)

Basic Profile of the Mother:

Name of the Mother: ....

Age: .... years

Religion: ....

Educational Status: ....

Occupation: ....

Register No.: ....

Obstetrical score:

G		P		L		A		S		D	

Date of delivery: ....

Previous contraceptive history: ....

Indication for intrauterine contraceptive device (IUCD) insertion: ....

Prepreparation of the mother: ....

....

Explanation about the procedure: ....

....

Obtaining consent form: ....

Preparation of the articles: ....

....

....

Specific instruction to the mother: ....

....

....

Types of IUCD used: ....

Procedure of IUCD insertion: ....

....

....

....

....

Aftercare and advice to the mother: ....

....

Remarks: ....

Signature of the Student | Signature of the Supervisor

Instruction: ....

....

ASSISTED FOR IUCD INSERTIONS (4)

Basic Profile of the Mother:

Name of the Mother: ....

Age: .... years

Religion: ....

Educational Status: ....

Occupation: ....

Register No.: ....

Obstetrical score:	G		P		L		A		S		D	

Date of delivery: ....

Previous contraceptive history: ....

Indication for intrauterine contraceptive device (IUCD) insertion: ....

Prepreparation of the mother: ....

....

Explanation about the procedure: ....

....

Obtaining consent form: ....

Preparation of the articles: ....

....

....

Specific instruction to the mother: ....

....

....

Types of IUCD used: ....

Procedure of IUCD insertion: ....

....

....

....

....

Aftercare and advice to the mother: ....

....

Remarks: ....

Signature of the Student

Signature of the Supervisor

Instruction: ....

....

ASSISTED FOR IUCD INSERTIONS (5)

Basic Profile of the Mother:

Name of the Mother: ....

Age: .... years

Religion: ....

Educational Status: ....

Occupation: ....

Register No.: ....

Obstetrical score:

G		P		L		A		S		D	

Date of delivery: ....

Previous contraceptive history: ....

Indication for intrauterine contraceptive device (IUCD) insertion: ....

Prepreparation of the mother: ....

....

Explanation about the procedure: ....

....

Obtaining consent form: ....

Preparation of the articles: ....

....

....

Specific instruction to the mother: ....

....

....

Types of IUCD used: ....

Procedure of IUCD insertion: ....

....

....

....

....

Aftercare and advice to the mother: ....

....

Remarks: ....

Signature of the Student | Signature of the Supervisor

Instruction: ....

....